THE
CORONA
TRANSMISSIONS

Alternatives for Engaging with COVID-19—from the Physical to the Metaphysical

A Sacred Planet Book

EDITED BY

SHERRI MITCHELL,
RICHARD GROSSINGER, AND KATHY GLASS

Healing Arts Press
Rochester, Vermont

Healing Arts Press
One Park Street
Rochester, Vermont 05767
www.HealingArtsPress.com

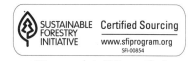

Text stock is SFI certified

Healing Arts Press is a division of Inner Traditions International

Sacred Planet Books are curated by Richard Grossinger, Inner Traditions editorial board member and cofounder and former publisher of North Atlantic Books. The Sacred Planet collection, published under the umbrella of the Inner Traditions family of imprints, publishes on the themes of consciousness, cosmology, alternative medicine, dreams, climate, permaculture, alchemy, shamanic studies, oracles, astrology, crystals, hyperobjects, locutions, and subtle bodies.

Note to the reader: *This book is intended as an informational guide. The remedies, approaches, and techniques described herein are meant to supplement, and not to be a substitute for, professional medical care or treatment. They should not be used to treat a serious ailment without prior consultation with a qualified health care professional.*

Cataloging-in-Publication Data for this title is available from the Library of Congress

ISBN 978-1-64411-307-3 (print)
ISBN 978-1-64411-308-0 (ebook)

Printed and bound in the United States by Lake Book Manufacturing, Inc. The text stock is SFI certified. The Sustainable Forestry Initiative® program promotes sustainable forest management.

10 9 8 7 6 5 4 3 2 1

Text design by Debbie Glogover and layout by Debbie Glogover and Priscilla Baker This book was typeset in Garamond Premier Pro with Trenda, Cache, ITC Legacy Sans Std, and Gill Sans MT Pro used as display typefaces

To send correspondence to the authors of this book, mail a first-class letter to the authors c/o Inner Traditions • Bear & Company, One Park Street, Rochester, VT 05767, and we will forward the communication.

CONTENTS

Royalties from this anthology go
to the Land Peace Foundation

"The soil you see is not ordinary soil . . . it is the dust of blood, the flesh, and bones of our ancestors. . . . The land as it is, is my blood and my dead, it is consecrated."

SHES-HIS – CROW

The Land Peace Foundation is a small, native-owned, Indigenous rights organization that is committed to the preservation of Indigenous culture, land, and water rights and the protection of sacred sites. We provide low-cost legal services, alternative dispute resolution, and training programs for Indigenous peoples and their allies who are working to build strong and effective Indigenous Rights Movements.

The five participating Wabanaki tribes are: Penobscot, Passamaquoddy, Mi'kmaq, Wolostaq, and Abenaki.

The preservation and promotion of the Indigenous way of Life includes the protection and preservation of Indigenous land, water, religious and/or spiritual rights; proliferation of cultural and traditional practices; strengthening of kinship roles; and preservation of ceremonial ways of being. The Land Peace Foundation provides a wide range of cultural, educational, and spiritual programs and is committed to be an objective resource for information on a variety of issues and concerns regarding Indigenous ways of knowing and being.

The Land Peace Foundation also works to facilitate the creation of enduring solutions to the ongoing threats of cultural genocide against Indigenous populations. Our purpose is to eliminate the likelihood that Indigenous peoples will be thrust into violent conflict; forcibly removed from their lands; stripped of their rights and/or resources; denied access and meaningful interaction with vital sacred places; and experience loss of connection to historical and emerging cultural practices.

CREATING NEW REALITIES

Richard Grossinger

Coronavirus Disease 2019 (or COVID-19) is the biggest event of our lifetimes, bigger than Hiroshima, the Asian tsunami, and the Islamic State. It arrived on the global scale of World War II but more comprehensively and discursively, for it is too tiny to defend against, too elusive to avoid, too swift-moving and eclectic to vanquish. It entered human history, ecology, and supply chains with the suddenness of 9/11. Though not as quick and stealthy a strike, its extent, duration, and toll have far exceeded a jihadist attack.

Ultimately, climate change will enforce a greater duration and toll than either 9/11 or World War II while joining COVID-19 in a futuristic matrix. Each is what philosopher Timothy Morton calls a hyperobject, a mixture of natural, cultural, and symbolic features that is vaster and more entangled than any cultural terminology or system can encompass. Together they form—and overdetermine—a hyperobjective Earth that is approaching us faster than we can approach it.

COVID-19 has created a new publishing category, perhaps the most instantly voluminous since Gutenberg. Some of its earliest texts were intended for the evangelical market and invoked God's punishment for the heresies and gender politics of modernity. Other books and articles proposed a homeostatic ecosystem trying to slow climate change. A coronavirus that doesn't kill everyone (like ebola or anthrax) forces us out of unexamined exploitation of Gaia and back into right relationship. Earth is not a dumb stone with some water, marketable minerals, and DNA fuzz but a living being that is part of our bodies.

Later texts addressed the mysteries and riddles of COVID-19, the hurried global searches for a cure and vaccine, and a new cultural, economic, and artistic order—more equitable societies and fairer wealth distributions—that might emerge from viral lockdown. QAnon-like fables sprang up in pandemic fashion, casting the virus as stealth biowarfare, political sabotage, a make-believe ailment with fake statistics, a meta-intelligent code or message from a higher intelligence, a Zen-like teaching from the microbiome, a socialist or capitalist plot, a poltergeist or haunting, debris from a comet's tail, or the advance weapon of an extraterrestrial invader. Threads of these float through this anthology, and it also offers more nuanced and hopeful approaches.

Before putting together *The Corona Transmissions,* Inner Traditions briefly considered publishing Laura Aversano's posts as a small book called *Love in the Time of Corona* (now excerpted within). By the time that idea had been floated, five other books using the same or a similar play on the title of Gabriel García Márquez's novel (*Love in the Time of Cholera*) had already been announced, the beginning of a burgeoning trope addressing a new world of social distancing, human contact, love, loss, and premature crossing over. Authors described homeless encampments on former pedestrian sidewalks, dystopian romances, murders of crows dominating cities and villages (flocks of these magician birds are called "murders"), herds of rats running down streets with the abandon of buffalo or lizards on desert rocks. The *Mad Max* landscape was medieval in its succession of panels: The Year of the Plague.

During an April phone conversation with Laura, I described a very bold crow that had landed next to me. She asked for an iPhone picture. I was too slow. She said, "He'll be back."

A day later, "Yes."

"Have you named him?"

Why, I wondered, would I do that?

Awaking in the middle of the night, it occurred to me, "The crow's name is obvious: CORVID."

Laura's email response:

"Wow . . . yes of course. perfect name for perfect medicine.
He is helping others to cross over but also issuing a warning,
there will be more to come, the earth is destined to purify one way
or the other, man is unfortunately making it worse.
Crow is acting like a psychopomp. I can relate—
Corvid the psychopomp,
as is the wind this morning."

Since everyone is sated with COVID information, speculation, and data, what is special and different about this anthology?

For one, it presents a wide spectrum of perspectives, from physical to metaphysical, from ecological to political, from apocalyptic to proto-utopian, and from scientific facts and health tips to imaginings, vision-ings, poems, and awakenings. Voices in the anthology address the virus directly, while others provide channels for COVID-19 to speak *to* us and *through* us. The virus is explored in terms of cultural critique, divi-nation, prophecy, warning, elucidation, and opportunity. It addresses our relationship to nature—to Gaia, to its animal, planet, and mineral kingdoms—to each other, and to the economies and dystopia we have created.

It also gives you vital hard-to-get information about how to prevent and treat Coronavirus-2019. This highly contagious life-form appears to be indefensible, as it throws a baffling array of asymptomatic states and dissonant symptoms and disease courses at the world. Yet potential remedies exist outside pharmaceutical and industrial tool kits. None are guaranteed, nor is there a one-size-fits-all solution, as there might be one day with a vaccine or wide-spectrum anti-viral metabolite. Instead, you will find here First Nations herbal allies and homeopathic T-cell boost-ers and nosodes. Cached in medical summaries, you will find anti-viral minerals, algae, vitamins, supplements, mushrooms, and anti-malarial inhibitors (both Western and Eastern) as well as sound, color, and light energies, thoughtforms, prayers, meditations, mantras, and affirmations that are indefinable in conventional materialist terms.

There is no explanation for how or why any of these should ward off or cure COVID-19, or any disease, but the same vitality that aggregates elemental molecules into cells, tissues, and organisms seems to flow creatively into biological fields from herbal essences, nano- and microdoses, the life energy of simple plants and stones, and our own subtle bodies and psychic fields.

The Corona Transmissions should be a welcome detour from the commoditization of COVID hysteria and clash. News media, politicians, and scientists, sometimes with the best intentions, use the plague to capitalize their own information systems, propaganda, and religious beliefs. In the guise of informing and preparing, they disenfranchise and disempower. They dilute our innate wisdom, diminish our capacity and resolve, and homogenize us for those who would exploit and imprison us behind rigid concepts, insidious paradigms, and obedience. Fear is a powerful mobilizer, the threat of death is its ultimate persuasion.

Our anthology asks you to respond, create new realities, resist easy categories and resolutions. Try to see through the hoopla and hype and receive your own vision. While reading these pieces, put the words of your heart and soul into the Akashic record alongside them. Send your COVID message to the universe. Make mantra, not politics. Transmit thoughtforms, catharses, and tonglen prayers. This book is just paper or electrons. You are spirit.

As a graffito chalked on the corner of Fulton and Carlton in Berkeley, California, put it, "Go Berkeley! Go World!"

Richard Grossinger's biography appears on page 371.

OVERVIEWS AND TRANSMISSIONS

TWO POEMS

KRISTIN FLYNTZ

AN IMAGINED LETTER
FROM COVID-19 TO HUMANS

Stop. Just stop.
It is no longer a request. It is a mandate.
We will help you.

We will bring the supersonic, high speed merry-go-round to a halt
We will stop
the planes
the trains
the schools
the malls
the meetings
the frenetic, furied rush of illusions and "obligations" that
    keep you from hearing our
single and shared beating heart,
the way we breathe together, in unison.
Our obligation is to each other,
As it has always been, even if, even though, you have forgotten.

We will interrupt this broadcast, the endless cacophonous
    broadcast of divisions and distractions,

to bring you this long-breaking news:
We are not well.
None of us; all of us are suffering.
Last year, the firestorms that scorched the lungs of the earth
did not give you pause.
Nor the typhoons in Africa, China, Japan.
Nor the fevered climates in Japan and India.
You have not been listening.
It is hard to listen when you are so busy all the time,
    hustling to uphold the comforts and conveniences that
    scaffold your lives.
But the foundation is giving way,
buckling under the weight of your needs and desires.
We will help you.
We will bring the firestorms to your body
We will bring the fever to your body
We will bring the burning, searing, and flooding to your lungs
that you might hear:
We are not well.

Despite what you might think or feel, we are not the enemy.
We are Messenger. We are Ally. We are a balancing force.
We are asking you:
To stop, to be still, to listen;
To move beyond your individual concerns and consider the
    concerns of all;
To be with your ignorance, to find your humility, to
    relinquish your thinking minds and travel deep into the
    mind of the heart;
To look up into the sky, streaked with fewer planes, and see
    it, to notice its condition: clear, smoky, smoggy, rainy?
    How much do you need it to be healthy so that you may
    also be healthy?

To look at a tree, and see it, to notice its condition: how
   does its health contribute to the health of the sky, to the
   air you need to be healthy?
To visit a river, and see it, to notice its condition: clear,
   clean, murky, polluted? How much do you need it to
   be healthy so that you may also be healthy? How does
   its health contribute to the health of the tree, who
   contributes to the health of the sky, so that you may also
   be healthy?

Many are afraid now.
Do not demonize your fear, and also, do not let it rule you.
   Instead, let it speak to you—in your stillness,
listen for its wisdom.
What might it be telling you about what is at work, at issue,
   at risk, beyond the threats of personal inconvenience
   and illness?
As the health of a tree, a river, the sky tells you about quality
   of your own health, what might the quality of your health
   tell you about the health of the rivers, the trees, the sky,
   and all of us who share this planet with you?

Stop.
Notice if you are resisting.
Notice what you are resisting.
Ask why.

Stop. Just stop.
Be still.
Listen.
Ask us what we might teach you about illness and healing,
   about what might be required so that all may be well.
We will help you, if you listen.

MARCH 12, 2020

You Can Touch Me
(AN INVITATION FROM QUARANTINE)

In the stillness of the house,
Loneliness is an uninvited guest
who occupies every room.
The woman's bright white terry cloth robe
suggests a cleanliness she does not feel;
the smells of disinfectant and burnt toast
hang in air that has the peculiar, leaden emptiness
of abandoned things.
The television is on, but muted;
facial expressions and body language
telegraph the state of affairs.
It is not good.
Her phone is silent but for once-daily check-ins
from far away voices.
This is by design, of course,
it is the nature of quarantine—
though the paperboy still waves to her through the window
when he tosses the day's news onto the front stoop
from a safe distance.
Her body aches with illness and lack of use.
She wonders when she will return to the world outside the
    window,
outside this room.
It is days since she has been touched
though she has felt the gaze of fear,
like a slap,
and the chill of isolation,
which like the fever, shakes her through the night
and sometimes, during the day.
"You can touch me," says the tree.
It is the hemlock, a low branch tapping on the pane.

She hesitates,
watching, listening.
"You can touch me," says the soil
from beneath winter-yellowed grass.
An invisible exhale rustles the hemlock's boughs.
"You can breathe freely with me," says the breeze.
"Come sit with me," says the great grey stone
at the edge of the yard.
With what remains of her strength
she pries open the window, extends her febrile head
like a bear cub emerging from its winter den,
or a turtle from its shell,
and blinks into a new day.
Brisk mid-March air soothes her scorched and weary lungs,
her eyes water in the sun.
The persistent ringing in her ears
becomes the song of a hundred birds,
Jay and sparrow, titmouse and finch.
The low hanging branch brushes her forehead,
its soft green needles tentative and gentle:
"Touch me, please.
Touch us and we will touch you.
Speak to us
and we will speak to you.
Let us remember each other,
Let us know each other again."

MARCH 13, 2020

KRISTIN FLYNTZ is a graduate of the University of Connecticut. Currently content editorial director at Ascensus, she directed Eve Ensler's *The Vagina*

Monologues from 2012 to 2015. During roughly the same period, she led high-school students at the Ethel Walker School in workshopping and performing excerpts from Eve Ensler's *I Am an Emotional Creature: The Secret Life of Girls Around the World*. Her objective was to encourage dialogue among the students and raise awareness in the community about issues impacting girls and young women around the globe while celebrating, supporting, and encouraging the gifts and resources inherent in young women.

ONE MORNING
DURING THE PANDEMIC

A Poem for Earth Day, 2020

Bobby Byrd

Revolutionary consciousness is to be found
Among the most ruthlessly exploited classes:
Animals, trees, water, air, grasses
—Gary Snyder

One morning during the pandemic
springtime
the city silent with the fear of death
a hedgehog cactus from among its dangerous spines
gave birth to a single luscious pink and white blossom,
the size of a man's fist,
its sexual core bright yellow and gooey—
"the promised one,"
as stated in the prophecies.
The blossom, once born in the sunshine, began to preach
    the gospel of the earth,
      its dance through the wide blue sky,

the sermon explaining
exactly
how and why humanity is not needed,
if it ever was, thank you,
for the earth, sun, moon and sky,
the great boundless universe,
to flourish
in the truth of love.
All day long the flower preached,
interrupted from time to time
by a pair of black-chinned hummingbirds,
seasonal migrants from south to north,
who kept coming by
greedy for communion, the body and blood,
take this and eat, take this and drink.
There was that one black bumblebee too,
squat little beast,
ravaging the delicate core of the flower's being.
The flower continued its sermonizing
unperturbed
while attending to these duties.
Neighbors and friends,
walking up and down the street,
stopped by to experience firsthand
the flower's message.
What they learned, only time will tell.
We'll see, won't we?
The flower preached until sunset
and during twilight it slowly
closed those delicate petals into itself,
packed its bag and disappeared
    forever. The cactus
    didn't seem to mind. It had small buds

already perched among its spines,
each with its own truth to tell
—in its own time, of course,
the long hot summer, the winter to come.

WEDNESDAY, APRIL 22, 2020

BOBBY BYRD grew up in Memphis during the golden age of the city's music scene. "That music," he says, "probably saved my life." Byrd has published ten books of poems, his most recent being *Otherwise My Life Is Ordinary*. He has received an NEA Fellowship for Poetry; the D. H. Lawrence Fellowship; an International Fellowship in Mexico funded jointly by the NEA and Belles Artes de México; and, with his wife, novelist and editor Lee Merrill Byrd, a Lannan Fellowship for Cultural Freedom. Byrd, Lee, and their three kids moved in 1978 to El Paso. In 1985, they founded Cinco Puntos Press, a very independent publishing company rooted in the US/Mexican Border. Byrd (his Buddhist name is "Kankin," meaning *sutra reader*) is the Abbott and lead teacher at El Paso's Both Sides No Sides Zen Center.

SUNDAY MORNING
SEQUESTERED IN AMERICA

Annabel Lee

I dreamed I saw the president.
He was walking through the streets
of Pittsfield, Mass.
There was no one out.
Everyone was at home
hungry and worried
about how they were going to
pay their rent.
My twin cousin came running up
to ask me how I'm doing.
I knew she wanted to know
who I wanted
to be our next president.
I was thinking about
the president right in front of us.
We walked through a grove of trees.
No one had been there in a long time.
There were a lot of dead branches
and the ground was littered

with debris.
We came out on to an ugly
Pittsfield plaza:
all concrete and empty
office buildings.
I shouted out, "People are
dying. Everyone I know
knows someone who's dead."
Secret service men appeared.
They surrounded the president.
"It's your fault," I shouted.
"You knew this was happening.
You knew more than we did.
You didn't tell us anything.
We weren't prepared.
You could have protected us.
And you aren't helping now:
everything you do and say
causes more people to die."
His big shiny van was
waiting. They all got in.
He'd heard me.
Night before last
I dreamed I saw Bob Dylan.
He was prancing onto the stage
like Mick Jagger.
The crowd went wild.
It was being televised.
I was in the audience.
Bruce Springsteen was on the
stage already: Bruce stepped away.
Dylan had arrived.
The master would sing the truth.

When I woke up
I made a phone call
to a loyal Dylanologist.
He told me Bob Dylan had released
his first new song in 8 years:
Murder Most Foul.
I listened to it all day long.
I wept because
the master was singing the truth.
A long time ago I dreamed
I saw the president.
Only it wasn't a dream.
The president was killed.
He'd been shot riding
in a Lincoln Continental convertible
through the streets of Dallas.
I saw it on TV.
First he was alive and then he was dead.
And at 2:38 the next president
was sworn in
standing in an airplane.
It was a magic trick,
just like Dylan said.
The rain is falling.
We knew it would.
In 3 days comes April:
the cruelest month.
The first day is for fools.
We are all fools and we wonder
why is this happening to me?
What did I do to deserve this?
What debts did I have to pay?

29 March 2020

ANNABEL LEE is the author of *Minnesota Drift, Basket, At the Heart of the World* (translations of Blaise Cendrars), and *Continental 34s*. Her poetry, prose, and essays have appeared in *Dodgems, Saturday Morning, Exquisite Corpse*, DianeRavitch.net, and in other journals and anthologies. She also translates poetry by Robert Walser and Louise de Vilmorin. She is founder and publisher of Vehicle Editions and a publisher featured in *Letterpress Revolution: Poetry, Art, & Typography* forthcoming 2020, Ugly Duckling Presse. She is the mother of Irene Lee, also a writer and publisher, and they co-published *A Book of Signs: The Women's March, January 21, 2017*, in its third printing. Besides editing and writing, she has been employed as travel agent, gas station attendant, real estate broker, art gallery director, executive director of marketing, driver, childcare provider, second-grade teacher, lighting designer, book designer, managing editor, production manager, printer representative, printer (letterpress and offset), bookbinder, and typesetter. A student of Tibetan Buddhism, her root teacher Traleg Kyabgon Rinpoche, she took the vow of refuge with the Karmapa. Formerly on the board of directors for The Center for Book Arts, New York, she currently serves on the board for The Poetry Project at St. Mark's Church.

LOVE IN THE
TIME OF CORONA

Laura Aversano

The emotionality of the virus began to shift this morning for the first time. Its consciousness is beginning to look at humanity in a different light. The collective energies around my clients last night and early this morning also began to lift. Its intentions are shifting as it settles more deeply into its "place" as an intelligent life force. My experience when this happens in this world means that it is in the midst of creating a relationship with our genomes, with the Earth, and in moving forward, our bodies, minds, the natural world will develop the capacity to handle this pandemic differently. I was waiting for the spirit world to show me a sign with the quieting of things beyond the veil. This might translate into emotions for us being very heightened this week, as when something this big begins to ground in such a way that shifts entire paradigms of existence, our emotions become rattled to the core. Find constructive ways of being in relationship with yourself, those you love, and life as we know it in the PRESENT. Allow for healing space to exist between you and the pandemic so your body and mind can respond to this crisis in the most healing of ways. (March 18, 2020)

◆ ◆ ◆

You are not feeling threatened by life. You are feeling threatened by the unknown. There is a difference. (March 18, 2020)

◆ ◆ ◆

All viruses have an innate intelligence.

They are as old as time itself and are a part of an ever-changing ecosystem that enters a host and attaches itself in various ways to cellular membranes as its genetic imprint forms a relationship. The way it will influence its host depends on many factors from emotional, environmental, spiritual, and through other epigenetic influences.

A virus contains DNA and RNA, just as we do. Its intelligence is far-reaching. It knows how to survive better than most humans do. It knows how to replicate, transmit, and cross boundary systems on many levels. From my perspective, their skill set is pretty impressive, and we could learn a lot from this living intelligence. Throughout history, we have created personal and interdependent relationships with viruses; and in my work for over 24 years, I have seen viral threads in people's epigenetic field, from their ancestry, still influencing current-day illnesses. I've also seen viruses react to certain frequencies. As times change, viruses and our relationship to them within our bodies change.

From a psychological and spiritual perspective, fear is a valid response but one in which a virus can also replicate itself energetically. I am watching how both personally and collectively, we as a society are dramatizing the pandemic. Don't get me wrong, precautions are warranted—but the truth of the matter is, viruses will exist until the end of time. Most of us carry viral threads and don't even know we have them. Many of us have been exposed to viruses from our ancestors and those viruses live in our bodies. My own great-grandmother died in the epidemic of the Spanish flu. The dramatization of any crisis comes in part out of fear of the unknown, our relationship to both power and powerlessness, and our ability to have a relationship with illness itself. Civilizations have faced pandemics and the loss of life since we evolved into being. There is a necessary life cycle for viruses and their counterparts just as there is for humanity. Hard to accept but all of creation breeds intelligent life-forms that might threaten our very existence. My own personal approach has been to have a conversation with the virus, as I do whenever I fall ill to a viral syndrome and find out what it needs from me and, possibly, what I might learn from it. A virus is not something in my belief that we can truly eradicate as a whole. They can be contained. There is a difference.

The environment we live in also plays a role in helping viruses to spread. When I used to do hands-on work eons ago, I would watch viruses in my clients run away from my hands. There has been research done on viruses being contained with higher frequencies of light. When Rife machines were popular, people believed in the efficacy of their frequencies to match those frequencies of many pathogens. Many living things in nature have high frequencies. Prayer has a high frequency. While the media is speaking of prevention, I am not hearing anything about how 5G, the overuse of pesticides, GMOs, etc., are contributing to weakened immunity and also the altering of DNA. Much of humanity enjoys an easier life unfortunately without consideration that our food supply, the air we breathe, technology, all impact our DNA on a cellular level. Thus, new viruses will be born and old ones will be resurrected. This is and will be the nature of things.

I'm sitting back, taking some precautions, but also opening up dialogue with Coronavirus to see what it has to teach humanity at this point in time. I also send my love and respect toward nature, for us not understanding or respecting the many forms of intelligence it breeds, wanting to eradicate anything that poses a threat that in the long run might serve us in ways we have yet to see. We cannot control the circle of life, folks. We can learn to be in relationship with it as best we can. (March 14, 2020)

◆ ◆ ◆

The Earth is helping us to understand the difference between entitlement and humility. The virus itself is learning the same lessons.

The energies being created through this virus will ground into the genetic matrix of both humans and the Earth alike, and years down the road, our bodies will have learned the lessons necessary to be in relationship with what we perceive is a threat to our humanity. I wonder if the virus feels as threatened as we do with its possible eradication? A living and breathing intelligence working to understand its role in the universe, its own relationship to humanity, and its relationship to its own survival. Entitlement and humility, a balance, one day, perhaps. (March 20, 2020)

◆ ◆ ◆

Isolation requires a tender moment of grace to allow yourself to continually feel part of the whole of the human experience, part of the whole of one's identity, part of the whole of all that is weaved through love. Be kind with your thoughts during this time of aloneness, judging nothing that is incomprehensible. Receive it lightly instead with compassion for what is deemed sacred will avail itself to you in times you least expect it. Presence lies within everything, especially in isolation, when you allow yourself to gently become one with it. (March 24, 2020)

◆ ◆ ◆

BEING IN RELATIONSHIP DURING THIS TIME

One of the greatest challenges that clients are sharing with me this past week is how to be in relationship with their partners at home. Jokes abound regarding the relationship lasting through this pandemic, an inability to foster a newfound spirit of communication, intimacy, reciprocity, emotional movement. The intensity and powerlessness of isolation create challenges for each person to learn to befriend themselves in a new light, let alone the person they share their life with. The trepidation of the unknown, the willingness or lack thereof to explore it safely and to hold space for another to do so can be overwhelming. Boundaries are shifting with each moment—physically, emotionally, and spiritually. Understanding the human condition at this juncture in time is not something we can wholeheartedly do, as the nature of the human condition is rapidly changing.

When we first enter into relationship, we are drawn by many factors, energetic conditioning being on the forefront inclusive of ancestral, emotional, and spiritual patterning. How we approach that conditioning will be influenced by the collective at this time in our lives. Most of us in this lifetime have not experienced a collective upheaval in planetary consciousness like this before. This will change our DNA to such levels that even the cellular memories of our ancestors will forever be different. Collective trauma and the way we relate to it will offer the opportunity for healing, in this world both for those who have come before us and for those who will come after us. As I write this, my DNA is shifting as a response to this pandemic, and how I looked at relationship yesterday is indeed different than how I am looking at it today. The same will be said for tomorrow. Our experience of love might change, as will how we work within that paradigm, how we communicate within that paradigm, and how we express ourselves. In these last few days people are truly concerned about being at home for such a long period of time with someone who all of a sudden feels like a stranger to them because of their reactions and responses to the pandemic and the fear. We are faced with surrender and compromise to such a degree that we fear the loss of an identity we have known since the time we came into this world. In doing so, we spiral into more fear, grief, anger, loss, and a plethora of other emotions that propel us into questioning who we are and who the person is we have committed ourselves to.

It will be important to establish physical, emotional, and spiritual "safe zones" within your home, with time allotted to become better acquainted with who you are during this great time of collective fear, hope, and transformation. The personal losses incurred during a shift like this can indeed be overwhelming and overpowering. How can you expect your partner to be clear about their relationship to what is happening when you aren't clear within yourself? The understandable power struggle that is unfolding right now within yourselves can easily be projected onto your partners. The word I am hearing from clients is a feeling of being trapped in the relationship. Love is there, but the everyday interactions of being in relationship have become so challenging that some people don't know where to turn. Circling back to various realities to respond to challenges might not work in the present. As much as we are all learning to respond to our reactions of physical isolation, we are all learning to respond to our relationship with emotional isolation, emotional exhaustion, and having to hold space for others in our lives.

Please be patient with yourselves and with those you love and who love you. We have entered into uncharted territory where the heart and mind are concerned. I expect you to be different when this is "over." I expect your relationships to be different. I expect endings and new beginnings. But we all have the choice to hold on tightly to these old patterns within relationship or head into the abyss with some excitement about the newness to come. (March 25, 2020)

◆ ◆ ◆

I'VE SEEN A GLIMPSE BEYOND THE VEIL OF WHAT IS TO COME.

A few of my clients this week asked about the future of humanity. Alas, wishing I were Goddess Divine and could alleviate suffering with one simple prayer, I did tune into the frequencies and saw glimpses of a parallel future reality that mirrored this one. (March 26, 2020)

◆ ◆ ◆

I do observe the natural world in response to what is happening. Living here in NY, a major epicenter of the pandemic at this moment that we know of, the energies are incredibly intense. I watch how my own animals respond and also watch the strays that I feed in my yard, the squirrels, the birds, any creature that will allow me to partake energetically of its behavioral patterning. Interesting thing to note is that my own pets are responding to my relationship with the pandemic, but I have not seen any of the outdoor animals respond as they usually would in times of panic, when something within the natural world threatens their very existence. I have spent a few moments each day, waiting, observing, and nothing out of the ordinary has yet to occur. I have set my feet on the ground as I do in times of illness upon the Earth, and again, all is quiet. The spirit world is a different matter. My mother who is an incredible "seer" will keep things to herself when she has a vision. She blurted out on the phone the other day, "This was all the death I was seeing." Death not necessarily in the literal sense. Its meaning encompasses many levels. The spirit world has been working tirelessly to help heal this crisis, assist those in sickness and in health, and be the light for those who transition to the other side. When I hold space for this parallel reality, I am in awe of the purification process that we are going through, wondering if the world has ever seen a shift like this since the times of the biblical flood. The intensity of detachment will render humanity stripped of a consciousness that was previously known. The waters are rising, and when this serves its purpose in the higher realms, we will come to know a stillness that we have never known collectively.

Until this comes to pass, we are all prayerfully doing the best we can to take care of ourselves and each other. (March 26, 2020)

◆ ◆ ◆

Social distancing does not mean we still can't rise together. (March 27, 2020)

◆ ◆ ◆

It's been a while since I've written a letter and felt compelled to reach out.

I don't know you personally, but rest assured my ancestors knew your ancestors both in times of great strength and in great weakness.

You have given me ample opportunity to pause and reflect. And for this, I am grateful.

My reflections have become so sacred and filled with gratitude for all that you are teaching me, all that you are teaching us.

I know you are in a time of exploring your own inner darkness as well as your light, and you have given humanity the distinct opportunity to do the same.

If your intention was to alienate and isolate human beings into a confounded state of oblivion, you have done the opposite, dear friend.

I have seen more stars at night yearning to come out in the day to guide us in our times of fear. I have witnessed more rainbows amidst the natural world as the Earth's manifestations take respite under God's care from man's recklessness. I watch as the sky settles into grace as the soil once again nourishes plant life in a way that it has not done so before. This rest you are providing us is regenerating the Earth and its inhabitants. Squirrels are dancing once again, trees praying in unison. Oh how I marvel at the miracles you have created.

You do not discriminate via race, religion, social status; my list could go on. How wise of you to share with us that grief, fear, anger, and every emotion under the rainbow embraces each of us equally. That suffering is inclusive, and not exclusive of identity or purpose. In fact, you have ignited an even greater purpose in our minds and hearts, and within the collective of the human construct. We as a world identity created such boundaries to keep us separate from one another, competing for self-worth and power, forgetting humility and honor many times. That is all changing now. We are beginning to see how those boundaries are self-limiting, self-destructive, and within themselves, foster an even greater sense of separation.

Even those who are beyond the veil are gathering in prayer and celebration during this time of evolution.

Tears flow down my cheeks as families spend more time with each other, relearning the art of communication and intimacy. Emotions once internalized are having a safe outlet to be shared. Entitlement is being humbled in dramatic ways. Love is being explored to such depths that we will come out as better human beings than we were before. Rest is being taken that never sees the light of day. You are showing us it is not us vs. them anymore, but us, just us. Finally. Tears again.

For those whose lives you are taking, they are so not alone as they transition. Our prayers have raised them to such heights that angels await their last breath to carry them home upon their wings. You have brought us many gifts, Corona, coming into our homes uninvited, or were you uninvited? Sometimes I wonder.

I wish you well on your journey to find the light.

And one day, perhaps we will meet as different souls on the journey.

Until you find stillness.

Laura (March 27, 2020)

• • •

Yesterday I needed to get out for some supplies and much-needed fresh air. It was raining off and on here in New York, a welcome respite from nature's tears to both replenish self and cleanse impurities amidst us. I took a detour to one of my favorite places in Westchester, a few towns along the Hudson River culminating in one of the most powerful portals I have ever embraced here on the East Coast. Many times, another sensitive friend and I have driven there to simply bask in its energies of healing and grace. One day as she and I were driving through one of the towns, we passed a burial ground, and I could not believe my eyes. Spirits were dancing amid the ground in large numbers, rejoicing, as though they had just been freed. I opened my window, as I could see them as plainly as I could see myself, and kept waving. I know it sounds funny but I had never witnessed such a mass exodus of souls from one plane/dimension to another in such a way. I have seen smaller shifts in the spirit world like this before, but something was different, something was very palpably different. They were free from their present state of manifestation and heading toward the next level of their spiritual destiny, and the leniency granted was so profound I just kept reminding myself of the prayers of mercy I used to pray for those departed who were stuck or simply waiting for familial miasms to heal so they might move on. Many traditions pray and hold ceremony for the departed to ask for graces and prayers from the unseen. If ever you needed a time to both ask for help and show gratitude toward your loved ones who are beyond the veil, now would be it. I promise you. Their prayers have just become all the more powerful. Amen. (March 30, 2020)

◆ ◆ ◆

And come twilight, the heavens will descend upon us with such a roar that all of creation will understand the miracles that have awakened us. (March 30, 2020)

◆ ◆ ◆

The lower levels of the spirit world are mirroring what is happening within the human collective right now.

The terror has become greater than the pandemic itself.

I feel like I need to say that again to offer the miasm some space.

The terror has become greater than the pandemic itself.

Please don't get me wrong. Fear is an appropriate psychological and emotional response to any threat or crisis. I am not going to ask you to replace fear with love. I just won't do that. I am going to ask you to hold space for both, to allow both possibilities to exist as you compartmentalize and internalize your reactions and responses to what is happening out there.

The fear has now taken on form, an energy form that is just as intrusive upon our boundary systems as is the Coronavirus. Even with social distancing, there are enough people in the world that no one has to struggle alone with this, no one. Even helping others through prayer.

We are all working diligently, respecting social distancing.

So what about enacting psychological, spiritual, and emotional distancing from those thoughts and reactions that are sending you further into the abyss?

There are things each of us can do to help ourselves and each other. The act of creation is our birthright.

The act and art of acceptance is also our birthright.

I see the light at the end of the tunnel.

I see the darkness even before we got to this place.

If we can create healthier relationships to our desperation, our powerlessness, our terror, we can shift some things here, everyone.

As human beings, we do not like to feel powerless. We have a hard time embracing suffering. We want to be in control of everything.

The paradigm of us vs. them can no longer survive in this new world being created, but we won't learn that lesson until we each explore our own personal relationships with power and powerlessness. Loss happens. It is happening. It will happen. We are each being faced with the loss of our personal identities, our roles in society, and the way we see others. Amen. What is on the other side of that has the opportunity to be miraculous, but that will not change the fact that much loss will occur. And with that, comes an intensity of grief and emptiness we have never allowed ourselves to experience before.

I am with you.

We are all with you.

May we cherish the opportunity to pray collectively for each other through these times.

Amen. (March 31, 2020)

◆ ◆ ◆

Sometimes the loneliest place is that pivotal moment when you lose sight of your inner strength.

Forged from grace, that strength is insurmountable by any illusion of fear that comes your way. (April 1, 2020)

◆ ◆ ◆

In this time of physical, emotional, and spiritual inconvenience, God is creating a new language for humanity, one in which we have the slightest awareness of the mercy that awaits us. (April 2, 2020)

◆ ◆ ◆

What an extraordinarily powerful wind last night here in New York City. I went out to bear witness to the magnificence of its purpose. A wind like that is deserving of such reverence and humility, as it carries souls from this world to the next. With rawness it carries emotions of those who have perished in this pandemic and those who are crying for their lost loved ones. Every tear is held in its powerful grace. Every anger soothed, every fear comforted. The wind is still strong this morning, fleeing from this world to the next with such swiftness, as called to by the gods of creation. I keep hearing the words, "Forgive us our trespasses." The heavens have given us such an opportunity during this time to explore our relationship to forgiveness—forgiving ourselves, those who have hurt us, and forgiving the unknown, the unseen, and a voice that has no name in our minds but is understood by all of creation. Thank you, wind, for carrying many of your children home. Amen. (April 3, 2020)

◆ ◆ ◆

MY LAST BREATH

I need for you to know I was not alone.

I could barely catch my breath. With every inhalation, memories of you would flood my mind, your smile, your warmth, our lives together. It made me pause, stripped away any fear I had about being isolated, waiting for that breath to fill me until I exhaled with relief. I knew my time was coming. You may not have been there, but everyone we know who had already made their way across worlds was by my side. I laughed as I watched souls reach for my hand to comfort me, some I had actually never even met. I knew they had succumbed to the same dire consequences as I did, part of this collective crossing of souls to such a degree that I am beginning to understand its purpose. Family members, friends, strangers, all in spirit form, gathered as I struggled for air and realized there was no way that any of us would ever be left to cross alone. The laughter emanating from these souls makes me forget the loud noises surrounding me from my hospital room, the machines I am hooked up to, the heavy energy and stench of fear that I felt when I was first brought here.

I'm taking my last breath now. I can see the angels parting those around me to reassure me of my ascent.

Oh, how blessed I am to be part of this calling, this mass evolution that will help heal humanity in ways I don't even understand quite yet. Their wings are so effervescent I can hardly contain myself. I'm lifting, I'm lifting. Boy, I wish you could see me fly. I wish you could feel how so untethered I am from everything that weighed me down. I wish you could know how many of us beyond the veil are praying for you all. What's happening to humanity is not what you think. I wish the angels would explain it to me so you would all suffer less until this has passed. But they won't. So I can't.

I'm sorry I left you too soon, but if you could only see this other world you would understand why. I am but a whisper away, helping you work through your fear of the unknown now and the plethora of emotions you are still feeling along with everyone else trying to make sense of the world right now. Humanity will be so different. The angels are jumping for joy at what will come. But I do know that a number of us had to cross worlds to prepare the way for you, and I was chosen as one of them. And just so you know, I would do it all over again because that is how much I love you. (April 3, 2020)

◆ ◆ ◆

Bless those whose enormous courage rivals that of any angel in heaven.

They are the chosen ones; those who have sacrificed their earthly experience during this time of crisis to enter into the world beyond the veil for the sake of humanity.

Their purpose is not lost, for it has finally been found.

Their pasts forgotten to innocence and humility as God awaits them at those heavenly doors, forgiving all misgivings upon their earthly embodiment.

They are the awakened ones, the ones whose prayers of hope and mercy will humble this pandemic until it settles into grace.

They are the awakened ones, the ones who will hold our hands in times of great fear and doubt, in times of despair and isolation.

They are the awakened ones, the ones who will unite us in a way humanity has never known before.

There is a purpose to their sacrifice, to their suffering, to our loss.

A purpose that we cannot explain or comprehend in our hearts at this moment in time.

But one we will come to understand as time passes.

Bless those whose enormous courage rivals that of any angel in heaven.

Humanity will forever be indebted for their passage of grace. (April 6, 2020)

◆ ◆ ◆

We are no longer standing at the threshold. We have become the threshold. Allow evolution to pass through you as gently as you can. Carrying yourself amidst the anguish of humanity, only to see yourself eventually rise along with it. And yes, you will rise. We all will. (April 8, 2020)

◆ ◆ ◆

Dear Coronavirus,

This past week has been incredibly intense and overwhelming in so many ways.

I've been excited to see the myriad of miracles you have been providing us with lately.

More so than when we first met your acquaintance.

I am hearing the laughter of children again, oh how they radiate such innocent joy in times of despair.

Spending more time with mommy and daddy, and siblings too.

Learning, embracing, feeling, hugging. I can't begin to tell you how many hugs you have ignited in our world. Even if some of those are virtual hugs at the moment, the love is so palpable my heart is bursting at the seams. Hugs within families, hugs between strangers, hugs that cross boundaries we once had that defined our separateness.

So many hugs I honestly want to share one with you, Corona.

You are brilliant in the ways that you have brought families closer; strangers are no longer strangers. Mothers are looking into the eyes of their children with presence, and fathers are tenderly nurturing what has been long forgotten.

Where walls once stood there are flowers blossoming everywhere!

You are teaching us so much about appreciation when much of what most of us lived by was entitlement.

I don't know how to contain my heart and my gratitude for your presence.

Your friend
Laura (April 9, 2020)

◆ ◆ ◆

You are the shelter you seek. In times of madness, and in times of grace. (April 9, 2020)

◆ ◆ ◆

Every last bit of healing medicine surrounding this pandemic will be passed down to future generations. Your children's children will remember how you responded to this time—physically, emotionally, and spiritually. It will influence how they respond in the face of crisis, and that in turn will influence their children. It's called epigenetics.

Let's show them what we're made of. (April 11 2020)

◆ ◆ ◆

I view Coronavirus as one of the greatest portals toward evolution of this century. Yes, many lives are being taken. But in truth, most of us are being given life. A life which we never knew existed before. An opportunity to love like no other and to care for humanity and the Earth in unprecedented ways. Embrace its teachings. (April 11, 2020)

◆ ◆ ◆

I AM ESSENTIAL

I am serving on the front lines now, putting my life at risk to save humanity not from a pandemic, but from the illusion of life itself you carry.

I have been essential throughout history, in all cultures, in all religions, all races, in every life-form that exists but you haven't noticed me until now.

You've only noticed me because you fear your life is at risk, but in truth, you have risked your life and the life of this earth for many a thing, most of which you call progress.

Well, that progress comes with sacrifice. Always has, always will.

Progress.

In the mid-1800s, thousands of Native Americans were forced from their ancestral lands in what is known as the Trail of Tears to make way for the "white" man.

The Tuskegee Study of African American Males to observe untreated syphilis so that those more fortunate could have the antidote.

The suffragettes.

Rosa Parks.

DDT pesticide use in American History.

Thalidomide.

History books can be filled with the sacrifices we have all made in the name of progress, in wanting more, needing more, in having more.

We have all become essential, or rather expendable.

How much more of humanity are we willing to sacrifice?

I hope it doesn't take another world crisis for us to notice how valuable human life is or the life of this Earth we call home.

Are our needs that great? (April 11, 2020)

◆ ◆ ◆

Enchained and shackled by fear.
Only to be freed by grace.
I promise. (April 12, 2020)

◆ ◆ ◆

Fearing the darkness might give you insight into your relationship with the darkness, but it might inhibit you from understanding your relationship to fear itself. (April 13, 2020)

• • •

Bless you, wind outside my window. I went out for a moment to feel your immense courage and strength, acting as a psychopomp, crossing souls from one world to the next. There are many souls in your bosom today, dear wind, so much so that when I stood still outside I tingled as they passed through me, illuminating my own etheric body. What do you have to teach me today, wind? Your might is fierce, perhaps even leaving behind some destruction in the wake of your path. But I do not fear you as your purpose is great: to raise these souls from suffering and bring them to the holy land of peace eternal. I do hear the confusion of those souls as they are crossing. I have been hearing it through my prayers this morning with clients. May their confusion and ours be comforted by faith, and by a warmth that only the Divine can ignite. When you hear the wind today, please say a prayer for those crossing. Your own heaviness will begin to lift. Amen. (April 13, 2020)

• • •

It is during this time when our innate sacred power will be revealed to us—a power that will exemplify a justice to be bestowed by the gods of heaven; one that will ignite humanity to cultivate a greater sense of compassion and humility more than ever before. This power will carry equal merit among every human being, leaving no one without dignity or grace, no one. We have been asked to carry this torch since time birthed itself into creation, but our own unworthiness instilled fear into our hearts and minds. This torch, this light for humanity, is indeed ready to be lit in ways unimaginable. Gather yourselves, gather your children, gather your friends and neighbors. The gods await our resurrection and the evolution toward a kinder, gentler, and more forgiving human experience. (April 13, 2020)

• • •

The collective trauma will continue some time after the pandemic. My greatest concern has been the long-term effects as we reenter our lives. There will be nothing normal about our reentries, as who we were before this time will no longer exist. We are in the midst of trying to figure out who we are now as we live day to day.

The compartmentalized reactions and responses to emotional and physical survival will avail themselves to us in various ways we may not quite understand; physically, emotionally, and spiritually. When individual trauma is bridged by collective trauma, it takes on form that needs healing and attention at a level that requires participation by everyone involved. It warms my heart to see humanity rising up to help each other, people reaching out to others in ways unimaginable.

During this time, if you can, gently grieve the loss of your identity and your role within familial and societal paradigms as you know it, readying yourself to be reborn. Because you will be reborn. We all will be. It is always a little intimidating coming out of that birth portal, descending into the unknown, a world that has the potential to be one of innocence if we choose to see it that way. I know I will. I know I will find the innocence amidst the chaos, the darkness, the purification, the loss. And within that innocence, a flower will bloom for all humanity. I can't wait. (April 13, 2020)

◆ ◆ ◆

In remembrance of the oppressed of every nation whose footprints walked this gentle Earth, help us to honor, oh ancestors, each suffering, each grave that carries the tears of those tormented by human iniquities. May their perseverance and might pave the way for humility amidst the human condition. May we be unburdened of false truths so that we stand together in compassionate unity. Those beyond the veil, forgive us for not understanding that your suffering is our suffering. That your oppression has become our oppression, that trauma repeats itself until we cultivate a mercy toward humanity that we have never known. Only then, will we be free. Amen. (April 17, 2020)

◆ ◆ ◆

Eventually, every darkness gets tired of running away from the light. (April 17, 2020)

◆ ◆ ◆

When this is over, you are not returning to the world. You are returning to yourself. In ways you could never imagine. (April 19, 2020)

◆ ◆ ◆

We are all being called to become epigenetic shape-shifters in this time in history. The past, the present, and the future depend on how we respond, react, and heal from this pandemic. Our cellular memory is being given the opportunity to heal its DNA in ways that will reach our ancestors beyond the veil. What has been coded in our genes is responding to our internal and external environments as I write this. I have witnessed such changes in the spirit world, from one dimension to the other. Boundaries between parallel realities are transforming. Many of you might notice an extraordinary sense of fatigue lately. With this much DNA transformation, rest is most certainly needed. (April 21, 2020)

◆ ◆ ◆

Oh great rain, your brilliant sojourn in this realm today left me speechless.

Dancing upon the Earth while whispering between the shadows of the ethers, you illuminated my senses with such purification

I can't help but contain myself.

I wanted to dance naked while each raindrop pressed against my flesh in sacred harmony; against a windswept backdrop of merciful revelations only the quietest of souls could hear.

I pray you let me dance with you the next time you visit, for you cleanse me of iniquities I no longer need to carry on this Earth. May your holiness become my holiness, oh blessed waters from the sky above. (April 21, 2020)

◆ ◆ ◆

And the tree whispered in my ear, "Thank you for remembering the sacred silence—this time of respite toward the Earth, with humanity standing still as we grieve together the pain of our world. We need this time to rest gently and to become acquainted with one another again, as equals under the sun." (April 22, 2020)

◆ ◆ ◆

. . . And as you surrender, the land beneath your feet will become Holy Ground, not as you have known it in the past, but as you envision it for your future and for those souls waiting to be born. (April 23, 2020)

◆ ◆ ◆

The vulnerable will rise to such great heights that they will be the new faces of evolution. (April 23, 2020)

◆ ◆ ◆

The ancestral keepers of the Earth are awakening in multitudes as humanity is stilled for a while. May their perseverance in mending the wounds of our home be given the time and respect it deserves. (April 25, 2020)

◆ ◆ ◆

Somewhere in between the ethers and the Earth our personal and collective identities become intertwined with the trauma unfolding within and around us.

Having an intimate relationship with ourselves is difficult enough without having to relearn this art with others. Our vulnerabilities become even more compromised, as does our personal space.

Our perceptions of ourselves, the roles we play within our families and societies, are responding to an inner and outer crisis where reality is skewed at the moment. Time is out of alignment for most of us; paradigms in which we have operated from emotionally, physically, and spiritually no longer carry the same weight as they once did. The illusion is for real. Hard to believe but how we see and value ourselves is changing with each moment that passes, and the person we see in front of the mirror may not be as recognizable. As we begin to experience life in new ways, our responses and reactions to those experiences, and to the emotions and thoughts surrounding them, will be different. They have to be or you might find yourself struggling more than you did before. How can we understand and appreciate intimacy when we can't even find our center in the midst of this global crisis? Looking at children or partners has some wondering, "Who are these people in front of me?" As though it is the first time meeting their acquaintance. What would intimacy even look like? How vulnerable a question.

Our vulnerabilities leave us teetering on the brink of power struggle. Our need for intimacy gets brushed aside as we concern ourselves with protecting the identities that made us who we are today. The thought of being without an identity leaves us empty, wandering the map of our souls in search of something that never really left us. The plethora of emotions that gets triggered projects itself into the many relationships we have formed and will also become internalized. Intimacy becomes scarce as we ravage the universe to fulfill a need that we think will make us whole. All the meanwhile, humanity could not be closer at the moment working through this crisis even though we are feeling so separated from those perceptions of who we thought we were. I am going to repeat that. Humanity could not be closer at the moment working through this crisis even though we are feeling so separated from those projections of who we thought we were.

Intimacy is taking on new meaning. Our need for it is also being redefined in ways we might have never expected. Our vulnerabilities are being challenged but so is our capacity to hold space for each other while evolution molds our identities into something greater than our prior understandings. If we try to capture the definition in the midst of a power struggle, we will not be successful in our endeavors and it will only create more stress within those bonds we hold sacred. The power struggle needs to be silenced for us to appreciate the dynamic unfolding within every person around us. Our needs have to be reevaluated. Our identities have to be abandoned so new ones may enter into the realm of possibility. Intimacy will happen. It already has. You just may not experience it if you keep holding on to the person you thought you were before this pandemic took hold of our world.

In grace,
Laura
(April 26, 2020)

♦ ♦ ♦

There are many who keep saying, "I'm waiting for this to be over." But "this" is where we are at now. What you see as confining is an expanse of human consciousness and the opportunity to forge new relationships with humility, oppression, and struggle—those same relationships that our ancestors looked upon with valor, integrity, with more acceptance than most modernized cultures of our world today. This pause is in our minds while those beyond the veil see it as a necessary construct toward healing. So no, I am not waiting for this to be over. I am looking forward to waking up each day and seeing how this is changing me for the better, changing us for the better, and changing the Earth for the better. (April 28, 2020)

♦ ♦ ♦

The rain is coming down hard tonight here in New York. There is no softness in its temperament. Its voice is so loud the echoes of what used to be are taking on physical form, compelling me to seek refuge and gentleness amidst the unknown. There is a weariness to its "voice." And as I write this, spirits are walking behind me through the portals that have been opening and available to all of us during this time. I don't know how many of you have carried a heavy heart this week, but some of those souls near to me are whispering words of regret, time lost; similar energies to the pounding rain right outside my door right now. There is one specific male soul around me, from long ago, connected to those crossing over during this pandemic. The others continue to "walk" by me. His regrets have become his identity beyond the veil, stuck in between realms, hardened by his earthly experience while here. I am telling him to cross with the others, to allow the rain to lift his bitterness so that his regrets soften and perhaps take refuge in a new realm of possibility. Refuge. Love that word. Whether it is refuge amidst the unknown or refuge in the pounding rain, may it soften us and all those regrets we carry until we meet that sacred refuge that lives within each and every one of us. (April 30, 2020)

♦ ♦ ♦

SHAME IN THE TIME OF CORONA

Shame has its place in our personal and collective histories. It has rooted itself amidst our vulnerabilities, more so today in our culture as most of us have never experienced a time like this before. Primordial communication existed between humans long before words were used. Emotions such as shame were raw in nature, hell-bent on wreaking havoc in our roles in familial dynamics and societies, and as it relates to how we see ourselves in this world. Shame is prevalent right now. This pandemic has triggered such a visceral response, none like I have seen before when it comes to this emotion. Whether it is shame of one's own fear around the pandemic, shame in working through the isolation, shame of contracting the illness, shame of losing one's job, shame of not being able to pay the bills on time or even put food on the table—an emotion that has separated us from time immemorial is now seeping into the hearts and minds of the collective at such a new level it is creating such a powerful miasm that our ancestors are rolling over in their graves.

Shame lessens our experience of life, our experience of one another, and our experience of ourselves. Our reactions and responses to life become muted in such a way that moving forward becomes a daunting task, as we cannot see that forest through the trees. The greater awareness of shame's purpose is not able to be reconciled within the choices we make, and we continue down that rabbit hole of self-deprecation until the shame becomes something familiar, something safe, something that takes away our authenticity and freedom. Its familiarity becomes a source of comfort in and of itself as we abandon any notion of worthiness, both human and spiritual. When we abandon ourselves due to shame, we reject our true nature and become stuck in that void of separation, unsure how to find our way back to the light. We then begin that search for power outside ourselves, seeking a false sense of protection that we think will help us function in this world.

I understand the reasoning behind the surge in this personal and collective emotion. I don't even ask that we eradicate it. It doesn't have to be as powerful as we think it is. It can be a tool, a very empowering tool, teaching us ways to step outside that power struggle within ourselves that has established an identity based on an unworthiness so deep that it causes us to act and think in destructive ways. We allow shame to take hold because our own worthiness is too great a risk. Unworthiness is an easier burden to bear.

What is happening to us does not have to create more shame. We are in control of how we emotionally relate to our present circumstances. Our fear, our anger, and all the other emotions surfacing as a result of this world crisis are valid emotions and deserve our worthiness so they can be attended to appropriately. Emotional freedom awaits each one of us.

May we carry each other through this time.

(May 1, 2020)

◆ ◆ ◆

AS THE WORLD SHIFTS

A whole new world awaits within you.

The heightened and intensified energies in our world these past few weeks have triggered ancestral miasms and memories to a degree that I have never seen before in my almost twenty-five years of practice. Cellular memories reaching out to me from those here and beyond the veil. Centuries-old trauma reawakening in clients, with voices wanting to be heard, voices wanting to be held, voices wanting to be healed. In all honesty, the exhaustion I felt spiritually these past few weeks was like none other. I heard the same from clients, friends, family. The push/pull between realms, crossing dimensions, expanding and contracting boundary systems on every level of humanity, individually and collectively, internally and externally. Many have felt an internal roller coaster and not sure when the ride would end or how it even began. Boundary systems are changing as we move from one reality to the next. The healing of ancestral collective trauma is painful. Thoughts, memories, emotions from ancestors of old manipulated by years of repetitive trauma, misunderstanding, oppression, injustice.

And when miasms become triggered so deeply, we begin to question ourselves, I mean really question ourselves. But our voices are not just our own. They can't be. They are our grandparents speaking through us, their grandparents speaking through them. They are trauma after trauma, memory after memory of wrongs needing to be held in the light. There is so much shifting in our DNA that it would be impossible to expect us to figure it all out now. There is too much confusion out there. Too much self-doubt. Boundaries take time to reconfigure— to expand or contract effortlessly between the light and the darkness, above and beyond any will we might have exercised to a greater will we are awakening to. This reconfiguration is actually causing a lot of physical symptoms for people, especially in these last few weeks. The confusion coupled with rage keeps a boundary rigid when the boundary needs to be given permission to expand into the light of the unknown, into the light of possibility, into the light of forgiveness.

So how can we forgive a wound? How can we forgive a trauma? How can we forgive a paradigm of confusion that has led humanity to think it is okay to hurt one another?

We begin slowly. We take each other by the hand as though each hand belonged to God. We take each memory and ask it to bless upon our hearts the forgiveness that we seek, the forgiveness we need to bestow. We ask those voices to pray with us, pray for us, and to allow us to pray for them. We bless each soul, one at a time, because we know that within each soul lies a myriad of souls, whose lives have weaved a tapestry of humanity that deserves the opportunity to know that the light can, indeed, overcome the darkness.

A whole new world awaits within all of us. (June 11, 2020)

◆ ◆ ◆

In the midst of this worldwide crisis, you are feeling everything unimaginable to the very core of your being.

You are being stripped of familiar boundaries in every relationship you have with yourself and with others.

Internal and external safety has become obsolete.

The rawness to which you are experiencing life is nothing many of you have known before.

Structures are disintegrating right before your very eyes.

People are changing and becoming unrecognizable.

You are becoming unrecognizable.

These wounds will change you.

They will change us all.

To be alive during this time, to bear witness to humanity and its involution and subsequent evolution is challenging.

But you are alive. You have that opportunity to recreate your internal and external boundary system with each passing day.

You have the opportunity to choose your reactions to humanity's upheavals as well as your own.

You have the opportunity to rise.

It won't be easy. There will be much more loss to come.

But you are choosing life.

And right now, this is where life is at.

For you, for all of us. (August 9, 2020)

Laura Aversano is an ancestral empath, medical and spiritual intuitive, and spiritwalker. Coming from a long lineage of seers, she has authored books on spirituality and healing, and serves an international clientele.

www.LauraAversano.com

WHAT PLUTO IS TRYING TO TELL US

Ellias Lonsdale

We are being visited by the aliens in our dreams who can be the aliens in our nightmares, who can be the aliens in the closet, who can be the aliens breaking out in the open and scaring us by how vulnerable we are to every kind of alien invasion we can live into. We are being checked out, and how we respond and react, as a species and individually, will determine much of our future, although it is primarily not a question of biology, it is a question of who we seek to become.

We know these deaths so well already. They have been advertised. They have invaded us to the point where we don't have an existence immune to them. The vaccine we are seeking would be an internal immunity, which comes when we are no longer afraid, when we are no longer in the market for finding our way out of here. In the stars, it's Pluto saying to us that the original impulse that got us this far on this planet has run out and that we are being required to fire up inside, to uncover a very different basis for why we are here. Pluto is not too concerned with our melodramas but is intent upon blowing up our every illusion and putting in place of it a void, an abyss, which we have to learn to cross without turning to our outer mind whatsoever.

The ego basis for existence is malignant. The soul basis for existence is unborn. The movement from old ego to new soul is what the species, and each one of us, is called upon to navigate. Time has run out. Time is running in. The world we knew is gone. The world we are going to know is here.

If we take it deep enough and subvert the authorities of mind, it is likely we will metamorphose from creepy-crawly critters into a fledgling species for myriad worlds to play through.

ELLIAS LONSDALE is a star-genesis innovator from astrology to cosmic reality. He is the author of *Inside Planets, Inside Degrees, Inside Star Vision, Star Sparks, Book of Theanna,* and *The Christ Letters.*

WHAT THE CELL TEACHES US IN TIME OF PLAGUE

Fr. Francis V. Tiso

In the sayings of the earliest Christian monks, we find those of the African Abbot Moses. A disciple asked him for a "good word": "Go, sit in your cell, and your cell will teach you everything."

This cell from which I write is on a hill outside the city of Isernia in central Italy. No one comes here. Many people go away from here, because there is no work. Very little traffic passes below my cottage in the hamlet of Colle Croce (the hill of the cross). The air is very pure. I can see a snow-capped mountain in the southeast, just beyond a ridge where the Blessed Mother is said to have appeared. That happened about the year my grandfather was born, just beyond the snow-capped mountain.

Officially, we are supposed to stay home. Go, sit in your cell, and try to keep this contagion from spreading. As I sit in my cell, I can see contagion in my own mind. The air is pure. Memories are not. It is a struggle not to condemn those who were not prepared for this epidemic. The older memories, though, are even harsher. The faces of those who hated me are like demons in a dream.

When the official decrees were issued, it felt like a shock. I was prepared for earthquakes. I was ready even for wars. An epidemic surprised me, even though I am well stocked with food and supplies. I have my herbal antivirals in quantity. For over three weeks, I felt a block against concepts and words. Anger took away my intelligence. It was strange to be made angry by the arrival of something I had foreseen. I could only do manual work. Then, slowly, ideas returned and I could begin to write again.

Then came memories. The real wellspring of anger was there. My cell was teaching me that I had not forgiven those whose faces like flickering candles smudged the walls while I prayed.

Again, the Desert Fathers advise: "Despise no one, condemn no one, rebuke no one; God will give you peace and your meditation will be undisturbed." With no one around, it seems easy to follow this rule. What about those who are far away, or even dead? Do not despise what they did. Do not condemn them for what they were. Do not compose rebukes against them. Recite the Psalms. Let the verses push those smoking flames as far as the east is from the west.

The Psalms are full of the notion of rescue from evil persons. The Psalmist seems often to be surrounded by enemies. Suddenly, rescue comes. Adonai can undo what human beings can do. Adonai gives joy to the heart of the rescued. Adonai keeps the singer safe. This is why we sing.

The early monks said: "Humility is yours if you forgive a brother who has injured you before he himself asks pardon." Forgive us our sins as . . . as we forgive those who sin against us. Before they ask, we forgive. Do we? Perhaps it is Adonai who forgives, especially when the smoking flames of memory prohibit our poor pardon.

Behind me stands a presence that does what my mind, weak in its stiffness, will not do.

In meditation, I drift off and dream. The Holy Mother from an icon I am repairing appears to me. She takes the Child close to her lips. She kisses it, over and over.

Your cell will teach you everything. When the faces of those who have hated you appear, you are being taught. A disciple is a pupil, a learner. The abuses of the past appear as soot and flame. You are learning. There is no one there. Still, you are learning.

You are not being asked to rebuke anyone. There is no need to condemn anyone. In any case, they are no longer here. You are alone. Except, the kisses rain down on your forehead.

In the past, your anger taught you to be free. Twenty years ago—in Tibet—that anger rose up like an eagle within you. Do you remember? You were learning. Someone was teaching. For two months, the signs of status were blown apart. In a state of utter clarity, nothing outside could menace. Nothing inside could disturb. Even now, should everything explode around you, kisses are what matters. We learn from kisses.

When two small panes of glass are pressed together, light forms a rainbow between them. The slightest motion alters the rainbow, made of waves of photons in interference. In the present moment, the world is like a dream. You can feel its dislocation and lack of solidity. Shift two fingers, and it seems like mist. Between the vapor droplets, rescue and pardon. Mercy is.

What we do for others in this particular time is not our doing. What we call compassion, or service, is not ours. If we forgive, we have only begun to learn. At least, let us learn. The future is given; it does not belong to us. It comes to us. And it will come. Everything is scattered; nothing holds its place. Still, we flow toward that bow of gratitude. Make of us an everlasting gift to You.

The anchoress Julian was taught to say: "It is true that sin is the cause of all this pain, but it is all going to be all right; everything is going to be all right." She was joyful in this revelation, and so are we.

April 2, 2020

Father Francis V. Tiso was associate director of the secretariat for ecumenical and interreligious affairs of the US Conference of Catholic Bishops from

2004 to 2009, where he served as liaison to Islam, Hinduism, Buddhism, the Sikhs, and Traditional religions as well as the Reformed confessions.

A New York native, Father Tiso holds the A.B. in medieval studies from Cornell University. He earned a master of divinity degree (*cum laude*) at Harvard University and holds a doctorate from Columbia University and Union Theological Seminary, where his specialization was Buddhist studies. He translated several early biographies of the Tibetan yogi and poet Milarepa for his dissertation on sanctity in Indo-Tibetan Buddhism. He has led research expeditions in South Asia, Tibet, and the Far East, and his teaching interests include Christian theology, history of religions, spirituality, ecumenism, and interreligious dialogue.

Father Tiso is a priest of the Diocese of Isernia-Venafro, Italy, where he now serves as chaplain to the migrant communities in the Province of Isernia. He is president and founder of the Association Archbishop Ettore Di Filippo, which serves migrant and vulnerable populations in the Province of Isernia. He was diocesan delegate for ecumenical and inter-religious affairs from 1990 to 1998 (re-appointed in 2016) and rector of the *Istituto Diocesano delle Scienze Religiose*.

In 1995 Father Tiso was invited to accompany Cardinal Francis Arinze, then head of the Pontifical Council for Interreligious Dialogue, to a dialogue with Buddhist leaders in Taiwan. He has traveled extensively in India, Nepal, Tibet, Thailand, Japan, and Bangladesh.

THE CORONATION

CHARLES EISENSTEIN

For years, normality has been stretched nearly to its breaking point, a rope pulled tighter and tighter, waiting for a nip of the black swan's beak to snap it in two. Now that the rope has snapped, do we tie its ends back together, or shall we undo its dangling braids still further, to see what we might weave from them?

Covid-19 is showing us that when humanity is united in common cause, phenomenally rapid change is possible. None of the world's problems are technically difficult to solve; they originate in human disagreement. In coherency, humanity's creative powers are boundless. A few months ago, a proposal to halt commercial air travel would have seemed preposterous. Likewise for the radical changes we are making in our social behavior, economy, and the role of government in our lives. Covid demonstrates the power of our collective will when we agree on what is important. What else might we achieve, in coherency? What do we want to achieve, and what world shall we create? That is always the next question when anyone awakens to their power.

Covid-19 is like a rehab intervention that breaks the addictive hold of normality. To interrupt a habit is to make it visible; it is to turn it from a compulsion to a choice. When the crisis subsides, we might have occasion to ask whether we want to return to normal, or whether there might be something we've seen during this break in the routines that we want to bring into the future. We might ask, after so many have lost their jobs, whether all of them are the jobs the world most needs, and whether our labor and creativity would be better applied elsewhere. We might ask, having done without it for a while, whether we really need so much air travel, Disneyworld vacations, or trade shows. What parts of the economy will we want to restore, and what parts might we choose to let go of? Covid has interrupted what looked to be like a military regime-change operation in Venezuela—perhaps imperialist wars are also one of those things we might relinquish in a future of global cooperation. And on a darker note, what among the things that are being taken away right now – civil liberties, freedom of assembly, sovereignty over our bodies, in-person gatherings, hugs, handshakes, and public life—might we need to exert intentional political and personal will to restore?

For most of my life, I have had the feeling that humanity was nearing a crossroads. Always the crisis, the collapse, the break was imminent, just around the bend, but it didn't come and it didn't come. Imagine walking a road, and up ahead you see it, you see the crossroads. It's just over the hill, around the bend, past the woods. Cresting the hill, you see you were mistaken, it was a mirage, it was farther away than you thought. You keep walking. Sometimes it comes into view, sometimes it disappears from sight and it seems like this road goes on forever. Maybe there isn't a crossroads. No, there it is again! Always it is almost here. Never is it here.

Now, all of a sudden, we go around a bend and here it is. We stop, hardly able to believe that now it is happening, hardly able to believe, after years of confinement to the road of our predecessors, that now we finally have a choice. We are right to stop, stunned at the newness of our situation. Of the hundred paths that radiate out in front of us, some lead in the same direction we've already been headed. Some lead to hell on earth. And some lead to a world more healed and more beautiful than we ever dared believe to be possible.

I write these words with the aim of standing here with you—

bewildered, scared maybe, yet also with a sense of new possibility—at this point of diverging paths. Let us gaze down some of them and see where they lead.

I heard this story last week from a friend. She was in a grocery store and saw a woman sobbing in the aisle. Flouting social distancing rules, she went to the woman and gave her a hug. "Thank you," the woman said, "that is the first time anyone has hugged me for ten days."

Going without hugs for a few weeks seems a small price to pay if it will stem an epidemic that could take millions of lives. Initially, the argument for social distancing was that it would save millions of lives by preventing a sudden surge of Covid cases from overwhelming the medical system. Now the authorities tell us that some social distancing may need to continue indefinitely, at least until there is an effective vaccine. I would like to put that argument in a larger context, especially as we look to the long term. Lest we institutionalize distancing and reengineer society around it, let us be aware of what choice we are making and why.

The same goes for the other changes happening around the coronavirus epidemic. Some commentators have observed how it plays neatly into an agenda of totalitarian control. A frightened public accepts abridgments of civil liberties that are otherwise hard to justify, such as the tracking of everyone's movements at all times, forcible medical treatment, involuntary quarantine, restrictions on travel and the freedom of assembly, censorship of what the authorities deem to be disinformation, suspension of habeas corpus, and military policing of civilians. Many of these were underway before Covid-19; since its advent, they have been irresistible. The same goes for the automation of commerce; the transition from participation in sports and entertainment to remote viewing; the migration of life from public to private spaces; the transition away from place-based schools toward online education, the destruction of small business, the decline of brick-and-mortar stores, and the movement of human work and leisure onto screens. Covid-19 is accelerating preexisting trends, political, economic, and social.

While the above are, in the short term, justified on the grounds of flattening the curve (the epidemiological growth curve), we are also hearing a lot about a "new normal"; that is to say, the changes may not be temporary at all. Since the threat of infectious disease, like the threat of terrorism, never goes away, control measures can easily become permanent. If we were going in this direction anyway, the current justification must be part of a deeper impulse. I will analyze this impulse in two parts: the reflex of control, and the war on death. Thus understood, an initiatory opportunity emerges, one that we are seeing already in the form of the solidarity, compassion, and care that Covid-19 has inspired.

THE REFLEX OF CONTROL

Gradually, the realization is dawning that health authorities greatly overestimated the deadliness of Covid-19.

Early reports were alarming; for weeks the official number from Wuhan, circulated endlessly in the media, was a shocking 3.4%. That, coupled with its highly contagious nature, pointed to tens of millions of deaths worldwide, or even as many as 100 million. In the ensuing months, estimates plunged as it became apparent that most cases are mild or asymptomatic. Since testing had been skewed towards the seriously ill, the death rate looked artificially high.

Every day the media reports the total number of Covid-19 cases, but no one has any idea what the true number is, because only a tiny proportion of the population has been tested. If tens of millions have the virus, asymptomatically, we would not know it. Further complicating the matter is that Covid-19 deaths may be over-reported (in many hospitals, if someone dies *with* Covid they are recorded as having died *from* Covid) or underreported (some may have died at home). Let me repeat: no one knows what is really happening, including me.[1, 2, 3, 4] Let us be aware of two contradictory tendencies in human affairs. The first is the tendency for hysteria to feed on itself, to exclude data points that don't play into the fear, and to create the world in its image. The second is denial, the irrational rejection of information that might disrupt normalcy and comfort.[5] How do you know what you believe is true? Cognitive biases such as these are especially virulent in an atmosphere of political polarization; for example, liberals will tend to reject any information that might be woven into a pro-Trump narrative, while conservatives will tend to embrace it.

In the face of the uncertainty, I'd like to make a prediction: The crisis will play out so that we never will know. If the final death tally, which will itself be the subject of dispute, is lower than feared, some will say that is because the controls worked. Others will say it is because the disease wasn't as dangerous as we were told.

To me, the most baffling puzzle is why at the present writing there seem to be no new cases in China. The government didn't initiate its lockdown until well after the virus was established. It should have spread widely during Chinese New Year, when, despite a few travel restrictions, nearly every plane, train, and bus is packed with people traveling all over the country. What is going on here? Again, I don't know, and neither do you.

Whatever the final death toll, let's look at some other numbers to get some perspective. My point is NOT that Covid isn't so bad and we shouldn't do anything. Bear with me. As of 2013, according to the FAO, five million children worldwide die of hunger; in 2018, 159 million children were stunted and 50 million were wasted. (Hunger was falling until recently, but has started to rise again in the last three years.) Five million is more than 100 times more people than have died so far from Covid-19, yet no government has declared a state of emergency or asked that we radically alter our way of life to save them. Nor do we see a comparable level of alarm and action around suicide—the mere tip of an iceberg of despair and depression—which kills over a million people a year globally and 50,000 in the USA. Or drug overdoses, which kill 70,000 in the USA, the autoimmunity epidemic, which affects 23.5 million (NIH figure) to 50 million (AARDA), or obesity, which afflicts well over 100 million. Why, for that matter, are we not in a frenzy about averting nuclear armageddon or ecological collapse, but, to the contrary, pursue choices that magnify those very dangers?

Please, the point here is not that we haven't changed our ways to stop children from starving, so we shouldn't change them for Covid either. It is the contrary: If we can change so radically for Covid-19, we can do it for these other conditions too. Let us ask why are we able to unify our collective will to stem this virus, but not to address other grave threats to humanity. Why, until now, has society been so frozen in its existing trajectory?

The answer is revealing. Simply, in the face of world hunger, addiction, autoimmunity, suicide, or ecological collapse, we as a society do not know what to do. That's because there is nothing external against which we can fight. Our go-to crisis responses, all of which are some version of control, aren't very effective in addressing these conditions. Now along comes a contagious epidemic, and finally we can spring into action. It is a crisis for which control works: quarantines, lockdowns, isolation, hand-washing; control of movement, control of information, control of our bodies. That makes Covid a convenient receptacle for our inchoate fears, a place to channel our growing sense of helplessness in the face of the changes overtaking the world. Covid-19 is a threat that we know how to meet. Unlike so many of our other fears, Covid-19 offers a plan.

Our civilization's established institutions are increasingly helpless to meet the challenges of our time. How they welcome a challenge that they finally can meet. How eager they are to embrace it as a paramount crisis. How naturally their systems of information management select for the most alarming portrayals of it. How easily the public joins the panic, embracing a threat that the authorities can handle as a proxy for the various unspeakable threats that they cannot.

Today, most of our challenges no longer succumb to force. Our antibiotics and surgery fail to meet the surging health crises of autoimmunity, addiction, and obesity. Our guns and bombs, built to conquer armies, are useless to erase hatred abroad or keep domestic violence out of our homes. Our police and prisons cannot heal the breeding conditions of crime. Our pesticides cannot restore ruined soil. Covid-19 recalls the good old days when the challenges of infectious diseases succumbed to modern medicine and hygiene, at the same time as the Nazis succumbed to the war machine, and nature itself succumbed, or so it seemed, to technological conquest and improvement. It recalls the days when our weapons worked and the world seemed indeed to be improving with each technology of control.

What kind of problem succumbs to domination and control? The kind caused by something from the outside, something Other. When the cause of the problem is something intimate to ourselves, like homelessness or inequality, addiction or autoimmunity, there is nothing to war against. We may try to install an enemy, blaming, for example, the billionaires, Vladimir Putin, or the Devil, but then we miss key information, such as the ground conditions that allow billionaires (or viruses) to replicate in the first place.

If there is one thing our civilization is good at, it is fighting an enemy. We welcome opportunities to do what we are good at, which prove the validity of our technologies, systems, and worldview. And so, we manufacture enemies, cast problems like crime, terrorism, and disease into us-versus-them terms, and mobilize our collective energies toward those endeavors that can be seen that way. Thus, we single out Covid-19 as a call to arms, reorganizing society as if for a war effort, while treating as normal the possibility of nuclear armageddon, ecological collapse, and five million children starving.

THE CONSPIRACY NARRATIVE

Because Covid-19 seems to justify so many items on the totalitarian wish list, there are those who believe it to be a deliberate power play. It is not my purpose to advance that theory nor to debunk it, although I will offer some meta-level comments. First a brief overview.

The theories (there are many variants) talk about Event 201

(sponsored by the Gates Foundation, CIA, etc. last October), and a 2010 Rockefeller Foundation white paper detailing a scenario called "Lockstep," both of which lay out the authoritarian response to a hypothetical pandemic. They observe that the infrastructure, technology, and legislative framework for martial law has been in preparation for many years. All that was needed, they say, was a way to make the public embrace it, and now that has come. Whether or not current controls are permanent, a precedent is being set for:

- The tracking of people's movements at all times (because coronavirus)
- The suspension of freedom of assembly (because coronavirus)
- The military policing of civilians (because coronavirus)
- Extrajudicial, indefinite detention (quarantine, because coronavirus)
- The banning of cash (because coronavirus)
- Censorship of the internet (to combat disinformation, because coronavirus)
- Compulsory vaccination and other medical treatment, establishing the state's sovereignty over our bodies (because coronavirus)
- The classification of all activities and destinations into the expressly permitted and the expressly forbidden (you can leave your house for this, but not that), eliminating the un-policed, non-juridical gray zone. That totality is the very essence of totalitarianism. Necessary now though, because, well, coronavirus.

This is juicy material for conspiracy theories. For all I know, one of those theories could be true; however, the same progression of events could unfold from an unconscious systemic tilt toward ever-increasing control. Where does this tilt come from? It is woven into civilization's DNA. For millennia, civilization (as opposed to small-scale traditional cultures) has understood progress as a matter of extending control onto the world: domesticating the wild, conquering the barbarians, mastering the forces of nature, and ordering society according to law and reason. The ascent of control accelerated with the Scientific Revolution, which launched "progress" to new heights: the ordering of reality into objective categories and quantities, and the mastering of materiality with technology. Finally, the social sciences promised to use the same means and methods to fulfill the ambition (which goes back to Plato and Confucius) to engineer a perfect society.

Those who administer civilization will therefore welcome any opportunity to strengthen their control, for after all, it is in service to a grand vision of human destiny: the perfectly ordered world, in which disease, crime, poverty, and perhaps suffering itself can be engineered out of existence. No nefarious motives are necessary. Of course they would like to keep track of everyone—all the better to ensure the common good. For them, Covid-19 shows how necessary that is. "Can we afford democratic freedoms in light of the coronavirus?" they ask. "Must we now, out of necessity, sacrifice those for our own safety?" It is a familiar refrain, for it has accompanied other crises in the past, like 9/11.

To rework a common metaphor, imagine a man with a hammer, stalking around looking for a reason to use it. Suddenly he sees a nail sticking out. He's been looking for a nail for a long time, pounding on screws and bolts and not accomplishing much. He inhabits a worldview in which hammers are the best tools, and the world can be made better by pounding in the nails. And here is a nail! We might suspect that in his eagerness he has placed the nail there himself, but it hardly matters. Maybe it isn't even a nail that's sticking out, but it resembles one enough to start pounding. When the tool is at the ready, an opportunity will arise to use it.

And I will add, for those inclined to doubt the authorities, maybe this time it really is a nail. In that case, the hammer is the right tool—and the principle of the hammer will emerge the stronger, ready for the screw, the button, the clip, and the tear.

Either way, the problem we deal with here is much deeper than that of overthrowing an evil coterie of Illuminati. Even if they do exist, given the tilt of civilization, the same trend would persist without them, or a new Illuminati would arise to assume the functions of the old.

True or false, the idea that the epidemic is some monstrous plot perpetrated by evildoers upon the public is not so far from the mindset of find-the-pathogen. It is a crusading mentality, a war mentality. It locates the source of a sociopolitical illness in a pathogen against which we may then fight, a victimizer separate from ourselves. It risks ignoring the conditions that make society fertile ground for the plot to take hold. Whether that ground was sown deliberately or by the wind is, for me, a secondary question.

What I will say next is relevant whether or not SARS-CoV2 is a genetically engineered bioweapon, is related to 5G rollout, is being used to prevent "disclosure," is a Trojan horse for totalitarian world government, is more deadly than we've been told, is less deadly than we've been told, originated in a Wuhan biolab, originated at Fort Detrick, or is exactly as the CDC and WHO have been telling us. It applies even if everyone is totally wrong about the role of the SARS-CoV-2 virus in the current epidemic. I have my opinions, but if there is one thing I have learned through the course of this emergency it is that I don't really know what is happening. I don't see how anyone can, amidst the seething farrago of news, fake news, rumors, suppressed information, conspiracy theories, propaganda, and politicized narratives that fill the internet. I wish a lot more people would embrace not knowing. I say that both to those who embrace the dominant narrative, as well as to those who hew to dissenting ones. What information might we be blocking out, in order to maintain the integrity of our viewpoints? Let's be humble in our beliefs: it is a matter of life and death.

THE WAR ON DEATH

My seven-year-old son hasn't seen or played with another child for weeks. Millions of others are in the same boat. Most would agree that a month or two without social interaction for all those children is a reasonable sacrifice to save a million lives. But how about to save 100,000 lives? And what if the sacrifice is not for a couple months but for a year? Five years? People will have different opinions on that, according to their underlying values.

Let's replace the foregoing questions with something more personal, that pierces the inhuman utilitarian thinking that turns people into statistics and sacrifices some of them for something else. The relevant question for me is: Would I ask all the nation's children to forego play for a season, if it would reduce my mother's risk of dying, or for that matter, my own risk? Or I might ask: Would I decree the end of human hugging and handshakes, if it would save my own life? This is not to devalue Mom's life or my own, both of which are precious. I am grateful for every day she is still with us. But these questions bring up deep issues. What is the right way to live? What is the right way to die?

The answer to such questions, whether asked on behalf of oneself or on behalf of society at large, depends on how we hold death and how much we value play, touch, and togetherness, along with civil liberties and personal freedom. There is no easy formula to balance these values.

Over my lifetime I've seen society place more and more emphasis on safety, security, and risk reduction. It has especially impacted childhood. As a young boy it was normal for me to roam a mile from home unsupervised—behavior that would earn parents a visit from Child Protective Services today. It also manifests in the form of latex gloves for more and more professions; hand sanitizer everywhere; locked, guarded, and surveilled school buildings; intensified airport and border security; heightened awareness of legal liability and liability insurance; metal detectors and searches before entering many sports arenas and public buildings, and so on. Writ large, it takes the form of the security state.

The mantra "safety first" comes from a value system that makes survival top priority, and that depreciates other values like fun, adventure, play, and the challenging of limits. Other cultures hold different priorities. For instance, many traditional and Indigenous cultures are much less protective of children, as documented in Jean Liedloff's classic, *The Continuum Concept.* They allow them risks and responsibilities that would seem insane to most modern people, believing that this is necessary for children to develop self-reliance and good judgment. I think most modern people, especially younger people, retain some of this inherent willingness to sacrifice safety in order to live life fully. The surrounding culture, however, lobbies us relentlessly to live in fear, and has constructed systems that embody fear. In them, staying safe is overridingly important. Thus we have a medical system in which most decisions are based on calculations of risk, and in which the worst possible outcome, marking the physician's ultimate failure, is death. Yet all the while, we know that death awaits us regardless. A life saved actually means a death postponed.

The ultimate fulfillment of civilization's program of control would be to triumph over death itself. Failing that, modern society settles for a facsimile of that triumph: denial rather than conquest. Ours is a society of death denial, from its hiding away of corpses, to its fetish for youthfulness, to its warehousing of old people in nursing homes. Even its obsession with money and property—extensions of the self, as the word "mine" indicates—expresses the delusion that the impermanent self can be made permanent through its attachments. All this is inevitable given the story-of-self that modernity offers: the separate individual in a world of Other. Surrounded by genetic, social, and economic competitors, that self must protect and dominate in order to thrive. It must do everything it can to forestall death, which (in the story of separation) is total annihilation. Biological science has even taught us that our very nature is to maximize our chances of surviving and reproducing.

I asked a friend, a medical doctor who has spent time with the Q'ero in Peru, whether the Q'ero would (if they could) intubate someone to prolong their life. "Of course not," she said. "They would summon the shaman to help him die well." Dying well (which isn't necessarily the same as dying painlessly) is not much in today's medical vocabulary. No hospital records are kept on whether patients die well. That would not be counted as a positive outcome. In the world of the separate self, death is the ultimate catastrophe.

But is it? Consider this perspective from Dr. Lissa Rankin: "Not all of us would want to be in an ICU, isolated from loved ones with a machine breathing for us, at risk of dying alone—even if it means they might increase their chance of survival. Some of us might rather be held in the arms of loved ones at home, even if that means our time has come. . . . Remember, death is no ending. Death is going home."[6]

When the self is understood as relational, interdependent, even inter-existent, then it bleeds over into the other, and the other bleeds over into the self. Understanding the self as a locus of consciousness in a matrix of relationship, one no longer searches for an enemy as the key to understanding every problem, but looks instead for imbalances in relationships. The War on Death gives way to the quest to live well and fully, and we see that fear of death is actually fear of life. How much of life will we forego to stay safe?

Totalitarianism—the perfection of control—is the inevitable end product of the mythology of the separate self. What else but a threat to life, like a war, would merit total control? Thus Orwell identified perpetual war as a crucial component of the Party's rule.

Against the backdrop of the program of control, death denial, and the separate self, the assumption that public policy should seek to minimize the number of deaths is nearly beyond question, a goal to which other values like play, freedom, etc. are subordinate. Covid-19 offers occasion to broaden that view. Yes, let us hold life sacred, more sacred than ever. Death teaches us that. Let us hold each person, young or old, sick or well, as the sacred, precious, beloved being that they are. And in the circle of our hearts, let us make room for other sacred values too. To hold life sacred is not just to live long, it is to live well and right and fully.

Like all fear, the fear around the coronavirus hints at what might lie beyond it. Anyone who has experienced the passing of someone close knows that death is a portal to love. Covid-19 has elevated death to prominence in the consciousness of a society that denies it. On the other side of the fear, we can see the love that death liberates. Let it pour forth. Let it saturate the soil of our culture and fill its aquifers so that it seeps up through the cracks of our crusted institutions, our systems, and our habits. Some of these may die too.

WHAT WORLD SHALL WE LIVE IN?

How much of life do we want to sacrifice at the altar of security? If it keeps us safer, do we want to live in a world where human beings never congregate? Do we want to wear masks in public all the time? Do we want to be medically examined every time we travel, if that will save some number of lives a year? Are we willing to accept the medicalization of life in general, handing over final sovereignty over our bodies to medical authorities (as selected by political ones)? Do we want every event to be a virtual event? How much are we willing to live in fear?

Covid-19 will eventually subside, but the threat of infectious disease is permanent. Our response to it sets a course for the future. Public life, communal life, the life of shared physicality has been dwindling over several generations. Instead of shopping at stores, we get things delivered to our homes. Instead of packs of kids playing outside, we have play dates and digital adventures. Instead of the public square, we have the online forum. Do we want to continue to insulate ourselves still further from each other and the world?

It is not hard to imagine, especially if social distancing is successful, that Covid-19 persists beyond the eighteen months we are being told to expect for it to run its course. It is not hard to imagine that new viruses will emerge during that time. It is not hard to imagine that emergency measures will become normal (so as to forestall the possibility of another outbreak), just as the state of emergency declared after 9/11 is still in effect today. It is not hard to imagine that (as we are being told), reinfection is possible, so that the disease will never run its course. That means that the temporary changes in our way of life may become permanent.

To reduce the risk of another pandemic, shall we choose to live in a society without hugs, handshakes, and high-fives, forever more? Shall we choose to live in a society where we no longer gather en masse? Shall the concert, the sports competition, and the festival be a thing of the past? Shall children no longer play with other children? Shall all human contact be mediated by computers and masks? No more dance classes, no more karate classes, no more conferences, no more churches? Is death reduction to be the standard by which to measure progress? Does human advancement mean separation? Is this the future?

The same question applies to the administrative tools required to control the movement of people and the flow of information. In some countries, one must print out a form from a government website in order to leave the house. It reminds me of school, where one's location must be authorized at all times. Or of prison. Do we envision a future of electronic hall passes, a system where freedom of movement is governed by state administrators and their software at all times, permanently? Where every movement is tracked, either permitted or prohibited? And, for our protection, where information that threatens our health (as decided, again, by various authorities) is censored for our own good? In the face of an emergency, like unto a state of war, we accept such restrictions and temporarily surrender our freedoms. Similar to 9/11, Covid-19 trumps all objections.

For the first time in history, the technological means exist to realize such a vision, at least in the developed world (for example, using cell-phone location data to enforce social distancing). After a bumpy transition, we could live in a society where nearly all of life happens online: shopping, meeting, entertainment, socializing, working, even dating. Is that what we want? How many lives saved is that worth?

I am sure that many of the controls in effect today will be partially relaxed in a few months. Partially relaxed, but at the ready. As long as infectious disease remains with us, they are likely to be reimposed, again and again, in the future, or be self-imposed in the form of habits. As Deborah Tannen says, contributing to a *Politico* article on how coronavirus will change the world permanently, 'We know now that touching things, being with other people and breathing the air in an enclosed space can be risky. . . . It could become second nature to recoil from shaking hands or touching our faces—and we may all fall heir to society-wide OCD, as none of us can stop washing our hands."[7] After thousands of years, millions of years, of touch, contact, and togetherness, is the pinnacle of human progress to be that we cease such activities because they are too risky?

LIFE IS COMMUNITY

The paradox of the program of control is that its progress rarely advances us any closer to its goal. Despite security systems in almost every upper middle-class home, people are no less anxious or insecure than they were a generation ago. Despite elaborate security measures, the schools are not seeing fewer mass shootings. Despite phenomenal progress in medical technology, people have if anything become less healthy over the past thirty years, as chronic disease has proliferated and life expectancy stagnated and, in the USA and Britain, started to decline.

The measures being instituted to control Covid-19, likewise, may end up causing more suffering and death than they prevent. Minimizing deaths means minimizing the deaths that we know how to predict and measure. It is impossible to measure the added deaths that might come from isolation-induced depression, for instance, or the despair caused by unemployment, or the lowered immunity and deterioration in health that chronic fear can cause.[8] Loneliness and lack of social contact has been shown to increase inflammation,[9] depression,[10] and dementia.[11] According to Lissa Rankin, M.D., air pollution increases risk of dying by 6 percent, obesity by 23 percent, alcohol abuse by 37 percent, and loneliness by 45 percent.[12]

Another danger that is off the ledger is the deterioration in immunity caused by excessive hygiene and distancing. It is not only social contact that is necessary for health, it is also contact with the microbial world. Generally speaking, microbes are not our enemies, they are our allies in health. A diverse gut biome, comprising bacteria, viruses, yeasts, and other organisms, is essential for a well-functioning immune system, and its diversity is maintained through contact with other people and with the world of life. Excessive hand-washing, overuse of antibiotics, aseptic cleanliness, and lack of human contact might do more harm than good. The resulting allergies and autoimmune disorders might be worse than the infectious disease they replace. Socially and biologically, health comes from community. Life does not thrive in isolation.

Seeing the world in us-versus-them terms blinds us to the reality that life and health happen in community. To take the example of infectious diseases, we fail to look beyond the evil pathogen and ask, What is the role of viruses in the microbiome?[13] What are the body conditions under which harmful viruses proliferate? Why do some people have mild symptoms and others severe ones (besides the catch-all non-explanation of "low resistance")? What positive role might flus, colds, and other non-lethal diseases play in the maintenance of health?

War-on-germs thinking brings results akin to those of the War on Terror, War on Crime, War on Weeds, and the endless wars we fight politically and interpersonally. First, it generates endless war; second, it diverts attention from the ground conditions that breed illness, terrorism, crime, weeds, and the rest.

Despite politicians' perennial claim that they pursue war for the sake of peace, war inevitably breeds more war. Bombing countries to kill terrorists not only ignores the ground conditions of terrorism, it exacerbates those conditions. Locking up criminals not only ignores the conditions that breed crime, it creates those conditions when it breaks up families and communities and acculturates the incarcerated to criminality. And regimes of antibiotics, vaccines, antivirals, and other medicines wreak havoc on body ecology, which is the foundation of strong immunity. Outside the body, the massive spraying campaigns sparked by Zika, Dengue Fever, and now Covid-19 will visit untold damage upon nature's ecology. Has anyone considered what the effects on the ecosystem will be when we douse it with antiviral compounds? Such a policy (which has been implemented in various places in China and India) is only thinkable from the mindset of separation, which does not understand that viruses are integral to the web of life.

To understand the point about ground conditions, consider some mortality statistics from Italy based on an analysis of hundreds of Covid-19 fatalities. Of those analyzed, less than 1% were free of serious chronic health conditions.[14] Some 75% suffered from hypertension, 35% from diabetes, 33% from cardiac ischemia, 24% from atrial fibrillation, 18% from low renal function, along with other conditions that I couldn't decipher from the Italian report.[15] Nearly half the deceased had three or more of these serious pathologies. Americans, beset by obesity, diabetes, and other chronic ailments, are at least as vulnerable as Italians. Should we blame the virus then (which killed few otherwise healthy people), or shall we blame underlying poor health? Here again the analogy of the taut rope applies. Millions of people in the modern world are in a precarious state of health, just waiting for something that would normally be trivial to send them over the edge. Of course, in the short term we want to save their lives; the danger is that we lose ourselves in an endless succession of short terms, fighting one infectious disease after another, and never engage the ground conditions that make people so vulnerable. That is a much harder problem, because these ground conditions will not change via fighting. There is no pathogen that causes diabetes or obesity, addiction, depression, or PTSD. Their causes are not an Other, not some virus separate from ourselves, and we its victims.

Even in diseases like Covid-19, in which we can name a pathogenic virus, matters are not so simple as a war between virus and victim. There is an alternative to the germ theory of disease that holds germs to be part of a larger process. When conditions are right, they multiply in the body, sometimes killing the host, but also, potentially, improving the conditions that accommodated them to begin with, for example by cleaning out accumulated toxic debris via mucus discharge, or (metaphorically speaking) burning them up with fever. Sometimes called "terrain theory," it says that germs are more symptom than cause of disease. As one meme explains it: "Your fish is sick. Germ theory: isolate the fish. Terrain theory: clean the tank."

A certain schizophrenia afflicts the modern culture of health. On the one hand, there is a burgeoning wellness movement that embraces alternative and holistic medicine. It advocates herbs, meditation, and yoga to boost immunity. It validates the emotional and spiritual dimensions of health, such as the power of attitudes and beliefs to sicken or to heal. All of this seems to have disappeared under the Covid tsunami, as society defaults to the old orthodoxy.

Case in point: California acupuncturists have been forced to shut down, having been deemed "non-essential." This is perfectly understandable from the perspective of conventional virology. But as one acupuncturist on Facebook observed, "What about my patient who I'm working with to get off opioids for his back pain? He's going to have to start using them again." From the worldview of medical authority, alternative modalities, social interaction, yoga classes, supplements, and so on are frivolous when it comes to real diseases caused by real viruses. They are relegated to an etheric realm of "wellness" in the face of a crisis. The resurgence of orthodoxy under Covid-19 is so intense that anything remotely unconventional, such as intravenous vitamin C, was completely off the table in the United States for several months (articles still abound "debunking" the "myth" that vitamin C can help fight Covid-19). Nor have I heard the CDC evangelize the benefits of elderberry extract, medicinal mushrooms, cutting sugar intake, NAC (N-acetyl L-cysteine), astragalus, or vitamin D. These are not just mushy speculation about "wellness," but are supported by extensive research and physiological explanations. For example, NAC has been shown to radically reduce incidence and severity of symptoms in flu-like illnesses.[16]

As the statistics I offered earlier on autoimmunity, obesity, etc., indicate, the U.S. and the modern world in general are facing a health crisis. Is the answer to do what we've been doing, only more thoroughly?

The response so far to Covid has been to double down on the orthodoxy and sweep unconventional practices and dissenting viewpoints aside. Another response would be to widen our lens and examine the entire system, including who pays for it, how access is granted, and how research is funded, expanding out to include marginal fields like herbal medicine, functional medicine, and energy medicine. Perhaps we can take this opportunity to reevaluate prevailing theories of illness, health, and the body. Yes, let's protect the sickened fish as best we can right now, but maybe next time we won't have to isolate and drug so many fish, if we can clean the tank.

We can use the break in normal, this pause at a crossroads, to consciously choose what path we shall follow moving forward: what kind of healthcare system, what paradigm of health, what kind of society. This reevaluation is already happening, as ideas like universal free healthcare in the USA gain new momentum. And that path leads to forks as well. What kind of healthcare will be universalized? Will it be merely available to all, or mandatory for all – each citizen a patient, perhaps with an invisible ink barcode tattoo certifying one is up to date on all compulsory vaccines and check-ups. Then you can go to school, board a plane, or enter a restaurant. This is one path to the future that is available to us.

Another option is available now too. Instead of doubling down on control, we could finally embrace the holistic paradigms and practices that have been waiting on the margins, waiting for the center to dissolve so that, in our humbled state, we can bring them into the center and build a new system around them.

THE CORONATION

There is an alternative to the paradise of perfect control that our civilization has so long pursued, and that recedes as fast as our progress, like a mirage on the horizon. Yes, we can proceed as before down the path toward greater insulation, isolation, domination, and separation. We can normalize heightened levels of separation and control, believe that they are necessary to keep us safe, and accept a world in which we are afraid to be near each other. Or we can take advantage of this pause, this break in normal, to turn onto a path of reunion, of holism, of the restoring of lost connections, of the repair of community and the rejoining of the web of life.

Do we double down on protecting the separate self, or do we accept the invitation into a world where all of us are in this together? It isn't just in medicine we encounter this question: it visits us politically, economically, and in our personal lives as well. Take for example the issue of hoarding, which embodies the idea, "There won't be enough for everyone, so I am going to make sure there is enough for me." Another response might be, "Some don't have enough, so I will share what I have with them." Are we to be survivalists or helpers? What is life for?

On a larger scale, people are asking questions that have until now lurked on activist margins. What should we do about the homeless? What should we do about the people in prisons? In Third World slums? What should we do about the unemployed? What about all the hotel maids, the Uber drivers, the plumbers and janitors and bus drivers and cashiers who cannot work from home? And so now, finally, ideas like student debt relief and universal basic income are blossoming. "How do we protect those susceptible to Covid?" invites us into "How do we care for vulnerable people in general?"

That is the impulse that stirs in us, regardless of the superficialities of our opinions about Covid's severity, origin, or best policy to address it. It is saying, let's get serious about taking care of each other. Let's remember how precious we all are and how precious life is. Let's take inventory of our civilization, strip it down to its studs, and see if we can build one more beautiful.

As Covid stirs our compassion, more and more of us realize that we don't want to go back to a normal so sorely lacking it. We have the opportunity now to forge a new, more compassionate normal.

As Rebecca Solnit describes in her marvelous book, *A Paradise Built in Hell,* disaster often liberates solidarity. A more beautiful world shimmers just beneath the surface, bobbing up whenever the systems that hold it underwater loosen their grip.

For a long time we, as a collective, have stood helpless in the face of an ever-sickening society. Whether it is declining health, decaying infrastructure, depression, suicide, addiction, ecological degradation, or concentration of wealth, the symptoms of civilizational malaise in the developed world are plain to see, but we have been stuck in the systems and patterns that cause them. Now, Covid has gifted us a reset.

A million forking paths lie before us. Universal basic income could mean an end to economic insecurity and the flowering of creativity as millions are freed from the work that Covid has shown us is less necessary than we thought. Or it could mean, with the decimation of small businesses, dependency on the state for a pittance that comes with strict conditions. The crisis could usher in totalitarianism or solidarity; medical martial law or a holistic renaissance; greater fear of the microbial world, or greater resiliency in participation in it; permanent norms of social distancing, or a renewed desire to come together.

What can guide us, as individuals and as a society, as we walk the garden of forking paths? At each junction, we can be aware of what we follow: fear or love, self-preservation or generosity. Shall we live in fear and build a society based on it? Shall we live to preserve our separate selves? Shall we use the crisis as a weapon against our political enemies? These are not all-or-nothing questions, all fear or all love. It is that a next step into love lies before us. It feels daring, but not reckless. It treasures life, while accepting death. And it trusts that with each step, the next will become visible.

Please don't think that choosing love over fear can be accomplished solely through an act of will, and that fear too can be conquered like a virus. The virus we face here is fear, whether it is fear of Covid-19, or fear of the totalitarian response to it, and this virus too has its terrain. Fear, along with addiction, depression, and a host of physical ills, flourishes in a terrain of separation and trauma: inherited trauma, childhood trauma, violence, war, abuse, neglect, shame, punishment, poverty, and the muted, normalized trauma that affects nearly everyone who lives in a monetized economy, undergoes modern schooling, or lives without community or connection to place. This terrain can be changed, by trauma healing on a personal level, by systemic change toward a more compassionate society, and by transforming the basic narrative of separation: the separate self in a world of other, me separate from you, humanity separate from nature. To be alone is a primal fear, and modern society has rendered us more and more alone. But the time of Reunion is here. Every act of compassion, kindness, courage, or generosity heals us from the story of separation, because it assures both actor and witness that we are in this together.

I will conclude by invoking one more dimension of the relationship between humans and viruses. Viruses are integral to evolution, not just of humans but of all eukaryotes. Viruses can transfer DNA from organism to organism, sometimes inserting it into the germline (where it becomes heritable).[17] Known as horizontal gene transfer, this is a primary mechanism of evolution, allowing life to evolve together much faster than is possible through random mutation. As Lynn Margulis once put it, we are our viruses.

And now let me venture into speculative territory. Perhaps the great diseases of civilization have quickened our biological and cultural evolution, bestowing key genetic information and offering both individual and collective initiation. Could the current pandemic be just that? Novel RNA codes are spreading from human to human, imbuing us with new genetic information; at the same time, we are receiving other, esoteric, "codes" that ride the back of the biological ones, disrupting our narratives and systems in the same way that an illness disrupts bodily physiology. The phenomenon follows the template of initiation: separation from normality, followed by a dilemma, breakdown, or ordeal, followed (if it is to be complete) by reintegration and celebration.

Now the question arises: Initiation into what? What is the specific nature and purpose of this initiation? The popular name for the pandemic offers a clue: coronavirus. A corona is a crown. "Novel coronavirus pandemic" means "a new coronation for all."

Already we can feel the power of who we might become. A true sovereign does not run in fear from life or from death. A true sovereign does not dominate and conquer (that is a shadow archetype, the Tyrant). The true sovereign serves the people, serves life, and respects the sovereignty of all people. The coronation marks the emergence of the unconscious into consciousness, the crystallization of chaos into order, the transcendence of compulsion into choice. We become the rulers of that which had ruled us. The New World Order that the conspiracy theorists fear is a shadow of the glorious possibility available to sovereign beings. No longer the vassals of fear, we can bring order to the kingdom and build an intentional society on the love already shining through the cracks of the world of separation.

APRIL 2020

CHARLES EISENSTEIN is a public speaker, gift-economy advocate, and the author of several books including *The Ascent of Humanity* (2007), *Sacred Economics* (2011), *The More Beautiful World Our Hearts Know Is Possible* (2013), and *Climate—A New Story* (2018).

NOTES

1. Philip Oltermann, "Germany's low coronavirus mortality rate intrigues experts," *Guardian,* March 22, 2020, https://www.theguardian.com/world/2020/mar/22/germany-low-coronavirus-mortality-rate-puzzles-experts.
2. Ruiyun Li, Sen Pei, Bin Chen et al., "Substantial undocumented infection facilitates the rapid dissemination of novel coronavirus (SARS-CoV-2)," *Science* 368, no. 6490 (May 1, 2020): 489–93, https://science.sciencemag.org/content/early/2020/03/24/science.abb3221.

3. Tina Hesman Saey, "Cruise ship outbreak helps pin down how deadly the new coronavirus is," *Science News*, March 12, 2020, https://www.sciencenews.org/article/coronavirus-outbreak-diamond-princess-cruise-ship-death-rate.

4. Timothy W Russell, Joel Hellewell, Christopher I Jarvis et al., "Estimating the infection and case fatality ratio for COVID-19 using age-adjusted data from the outbreak on the Diamond Princess cruise ship," *Eurosurveillance* 25, no. 12 (March 26, 2020), https://www.eurosurveillance.org/content/10.2807/1560-7917.ES.2020.25.12.2000256.

5. *Encyclopaedia Britannica Online*, s.v. "1968 flu pandemic," by Kara Rogers, last modified March 25, 2020, https://www.britannica.com/event/1968-flu-pandemic.

5. Daniel Schmachtenberger, "Mind viruses during a pandemic:," Facebook page, March 17, 2020, https://m.facebook.com/notes/daniel-schmachtenberger/mind-viruses-during-a-pandemic/10156663879545213/.

6. https://www.facebook.com/search/top/?q=lissa%20rankin

7. *Politico* Magazine, "Coronavirus Will Change the World Permanently. Here's How," March 19, 2020, https://www.politico.com/news/magazine/2020/03/19/coronavirus-effect-economy-life-society-analysis-covid-135579.

8. Jaime Rosenberg, "The Effects of Chronic Fear on a Person's Health," *AJMC*, November 11, 2017, https://www.ajmc.com/conferences/nei-2017/the-effects-of-chronic-fear-on-a-persons-health.

9. Steven W. Cole et al., "Myeloid differentiation architecture of leukocyte transcriptome dynamics in perceived social isolation," *PNAS* 112, no. 49 (December 8, 2015): 15142–47, https://www.pnas.org/content/112/49/15142.

10. Alice G. Walton, "7 Ways Loneliness (and Connectedness) Affect Mental Health," *Forbes,* October 30, 2018, https://www.forbes.com/sites/alicegwalton/2018/10/30/7-ways-loneliness-and-connectedness-affect-mental-health/#6297c37ce1dc.

11. Kate Anderton, ed., "Social contact could play an important role in staving off dementia," *News Medical,* August 3, 2019, https://www.news-medical.net/news/20190803/Social-contact-could-play-an-important-role-in-staving-off-dementia.aspx.

12. Lissa Rankin, "The #1 Public Health Issue Doctors Aren't Talking About," TEDxFargo, September 28, 2016, YouTube video, https://www.youtube.com/watch?v=s2hLhWSlOl0.

13. Herbert W. 'Skip' Virgin IV, "The mammalian virome in genetic analysis

of health and disease pathogenesis," R. E. Dyer lecture, National Institutes of Health, streamed live on April 22, 2015, YouTube video, https://www .youtube.com/watch?v=TRVxTBuvChU.

14. Tommaso Ebhardt, Chiara Remondini, and Marco Bertacche, "99% of Those Who Died From Virus Had Other Illness, Italy Says," *Bloomberg,* March 18, 2020, https://www.bloomberg.com/news/articles/2020-03-18/99-of-those-who-died-from-virus-had-other-illness-italy-says.

15. "Report sulle caratteristiche dei pazienti deceduti positivi a COVID-19 in Italia," *EpiCentro,* Istituto Superiore di Sanitá, March 17, 2020, https:// www.epicentro.iss.it/coronavirus/bollettino/Report-COVID-2019_17_ marzo-v2.pdf.

16. S. De Flora, C. Grassi, and L. Carati, "Attenuation of influenza-like symp- tomatology and improvement of cell-mediated immunity with long-term N-acetylcysteine treatment," *European Respiratory Journal* 10, no. 7 (July 1, 1997): 1535–41, https://erj.ersjournals.com/content/10/7/1535.long.

17. Brig Klyce, "Viruses and Other Gene Transfer Mechanisms," *Cosmic Ancestry* (blog), Astrobiology Research Trust, https://www.panspermia.org /virus.htm.

AN APPROPRIATE RESPONSE

Reconnecting the Dots

GARY GACH

We will not go back to normal. Normal never was. Our pre-corona existence was not normal other than we normalized greed, inequity, exhaustion, depletion, extraction, disconnection, confusion, rage, hoarding, hate, and lack. We should not long to return, my friends. We are being given the opportunity to stitch a new garment. One that fits all of humanity and nature.

—SONYA RENEE TAYLOR[1]

SPRINGING INTO PARADIGM SHIFTING

This pandemic feels like winter. Yet around me I see ginkgo trees sprouting leaves and cherry trees blooming. So I recognize and accept this pandemic has begun in spring, season of new ideas. Pulling all the sheets to its side of the bed, as it were, it certainly seems to recontextualize everything.

To speak of it as a crisis conforms to the Middle English usage of the word as "the decisive point in the progress of a disease." On the other hand, there's a common misconception that the Chinese word for "crisis" is composed of characters for "danger" and "opportunity," but it's a useful misconception nevertheless. In a crisis everything not nailed down is shaking loose. The positive side of that is how what was once seen as impossible can become reality.

Be on the look-out. In times when an outworn working model is transforming into a new one, all sorts of proposals and ideas previously shelved can get dusted off for reconsideration and possible application.

Be careful too. A time of paradigm shift can also be one of power shift, as Naomi Klein has soberly laid out in her theory of shock doctrine.

As always, cleave to the middle way. The neat part of that is locating the middle path in any situation. Not a straight and narrow path, it's always changing, like a river. The Taoist diagram shows it clearly.

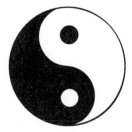

MY COLLEGE IMMUNOLOGY TEXTBOOK

I'm over 70. So I'm automatically enrolled in the death demographic of COVID-19 epidemiology. In lieu of a vaccine, my fate could well boil down to the health of my immune system. So I've been brushing up on immunology.

I remember when I studied physiology in college, in the late 1960s. At the time, the class was told that immunology is a newcomer to our studies of human bodily systems. It didn't begin to coalesce until the mid-1950s–1960s, with the discovery of cytokines and the role of the thymus, the structure of antibodies, the interaction of T-cells and B-cells, humoral vs. cellular immunology, and so on.

Looking at it now, it's key to see how immunology's era of initial recognition shines a light and casts a shadow on our current understanding.

(If immunology is a living system, we can explore its relation to its environment as an immunological study.) Coming together as a major discipline during the tragic U.S. war in Vietnam, immunology is deeply rooted in military soil. Immunological response, as we know it today, is framed in terms of defense and attack, self vs. other, Us vs. Them, search and destroy. This, in turn, is anchored in a dualist paradigm, inherited from the philosophy of Aristotle and Descartes.

Fortunately, there are viable non-military, non-dualist models yet to be embraced. Here follows just one such avenue for further research and application.

IMMU-KNOWLEDGE

The present need of immunology is not merely to discover new molecular building-blocks; at this stage we have an abundance, perhaps even a glut, of basic molecules. We now need to understand the ways the molecules interact to create a system . . . . Confounded by its very success, immunology finds itself in need of new unifying ideas, a new paradigm.

—Irun Cohen, *Tending Adam's Garden: Evolving the Cognitive Immune System*

Mathematician, biologist, neurophenomenologist Francisco Varela has studied immunology for a decade. If I might shoehorn a sleeve of his studies into a few paragraphs, I'd begin by saying it's more about how an organism defines and redefines itself throughout its lifetime, through interacting with its environment, rather than how it defends itself from shock invasions. Taking flight-fight-or-freeze as our normal baseline, for example, relegates consciousness to that portion of our brain we inherited from dinosaurs, sitting on the end of the spine.

Similarly, to say that human immunology is a defense system is like saying Earth's ecosystems evolved because of meteors. The Earth can cope with meteors, but they're freak events, as is COVID-19. These are exceptions from the symbiotic network of chemical reactions and interactions that comprise normal immunological processes. Massive inflammation as an immune response can compromise the body's integrity. So too the "cytokine storm" of COVID-19, where the body initiates massive immune response, is what is fatal, not the virus itself. These are both abnormal circumstances.

From birth, an invertebrate has a range of chemical substances with which to define itself. When new chemicals enter the system, these substances can modify the body's chemicals, the modified innate chemicals then modify the system, and together they mutually become part of the evolving living system.

A useful neologism here is *autopoiesis:* the ability of living organisms to self-regulate their composition and boundaries. The ability of all living beings—"from bacterial speck, to congressional committee member"—to exempt themselves from disease is autopoietic. As such, it's a mode of cognition, emergent from the interrelationships of a community of molecules. This view allows for our interaction with our environment as a mutual awakening.

Looking deeper, it all comes back to Mother Earth. I touch my hand, it is Mother Earth touching Mother Earth. We are each Mother Earth, walking on Mother Earth, walking each other back home.

GAIAN SCIENCE

Harking back to the Darwinian paradigm of evolution, we can see how it implies a fierce competition between isolated species: "nature red in tooth and claw." But more recently microbiologist Lynn Margulis uncovered how evolution is indebted to the interactive, cooperative symbiosis among different life-forms. That is, while Darwin conceived of nature as a static, fixed environment, Lynn Margulis showed how organisms and their environment are in a constant state of co-evolution. (We make the road, and the road makes us.)

Her groundbreaking work shook loose two other standard scientific assumptions. Her research also revealed life's basic building block—the cell—to be a symbiotic merger of different varieties of bacteria. Following along these lines—seeing both the cell and evolution as interactive processes—with James Lovelock, she hypothesized that Earth herself is a living being. (Call her "Gaia.") In other words, all organisms to which she gives birth are elements of the interaction of her organic and inorganic environments, creating a complex, self-regulating, synergistic, living system.

GOING VIRAL & HEEDING THE CALL

Reframing the COVID-19 crisis in the light of Gaian evolution, I take a step back. I recall how our epoch, following the Holocene, has been called by many the "Anthropocene." That means human impact on Earth's biosphere now rivals previous natural agents of change, such as asteroid collision, advance of ice sheets, new species on the scene, and so on. Our cognitive processes have now become planetary processes. The light of COVID-19 invites me to pause and reflect on a major vehicle of our contemporary cognitive processes.

Our society's already been drifting, since mid-century, from the traditional marriage of science and technology, to an emphasis on technology (science as engineering), which now features the digital and the virtual. Mid-April (2020), I'm hearing how this pandemic might hasten the widespread adoption of computer-related, virtual culture. Is it a good thing? Well, connect the dots.

Computer culture certainly spreads like a virus. Seen under the microscope, a virus shows many lifelike properties. Yet it's dependent on a host for life and growth. It may mutate, yet it's not capable of natural regeneration, the way roots and branches can seasonally devote all their energy to blossoming.

Consider too that the structure of a virus is crystalline. And a virus shares a basic morphology with computers, whose primary building block—silicon—is also crystalline. At its best, the crystalline quality of computer culture reflects our ancient wisdom traditions' profound insight as to the internetworked nature of reality (the image of Indra's net of jewels, for instance). Yet with everything on the inter-web being facets equidistant from each other, values seem more and more relative. And along with such growing post-Modernist relativism comes a sense of isolation. A grounded trunk of roots and branches morphs into an ever-lengthening tail of isolated nodes.

This isn't a solely intellectual construct. Walking around my hill in San Francisco—to commune with nature, absorb sunshine, and exercise—I have to give wide berth to strangers walking along alone in conversation with their invisible, virtual friend, ears plugged into silicon phones, oblivious to real people on the actual sidewalk. And I see otherwise empty cars with drivers wearing a mask, windows rolled up.

Hello?

This, in turn, reminds me how, as a means of communication, as now a public address system, digital culture has accelerated the globalization of our planet. Activating my historical memory again, I recall how the porosity of borders during the globalization of the Mongol Empire facilitated the transmission of deadly bacilli that resulted in the devastating Bubonic Plague. Will we reconceive globalization, and culture, in light of COVID-19?

One more phenomenon from the Mongol Empire comes to mind, before I seek closure. When Marco Polo visited China, he was impressed by the Mongols' use of paper (rather than metal) currency. He called it one of the wonders of the world. But, easy to print, it also led to runaway inflation, which led to income disparity, which ultimately helped spell the demise of the Empire.

Today, the dominant US economic model seems to say there is no deficit, and money can be printed at will. But one life-form that resembles an economy based on unlimited growth is: cancer. Like a virus, cancer can, if not checked in time, destroy its host environment.

Environmental degradation is one big indicator. As we confront the growing economic havoc COVID-19 is sure to wreak, may we learn how to hear the *eco* in economy as well as ecology?

Can we heed the call? COVID-19 brings us to a remarkable crossroads. Remembering Gaian wisdom, as self-aware beings within a living ecosphere, is it possible we may be a portal through which the cosmos is awakening to its own self-awareness? Or might Mother Earth consider us too dangerous a virus? Might she flick us off her back, making room for other, more adaptive life-forms to inhabit her blue-green ecosphere in co-evolutionary, homeostatic, symbiotic harmony and balance? And might our realizing this possibility be itself a moment of a great awakening?

WAKING UP IN THE WORLD

In the unfolding diplomacy of events—what is an appropriate response? Connecting these initial dots, I've begun to improvise a star chart by which to steer. I'd like to wrap up here with just a couple more dots— noble, needful, vital dots.

In my ongoing studies, observations, and practice—to recognize, understand, and embrace the nonpersonal, ever-provisional, permeable nature of reality is always fundamental. COVID-19 sure raises the ante.

The impersonal nature of things grants me a spaciousness of view— a bigger container than what Alan Watts called "the skin-encapsulated ego." Lately, I call this view "equanimity." That's inclusive of the peace, joy, and loving I know from looking directly at What Is. Recognizing things are how they are helps me both remain calm in emergency and be poised for action in the midst of calm. It also engenders a continual curiosity: what is *this*?

I find impermanence training my resilience, oh so needful today. Having already included impermanence on my watch list, when it comes on in a big way, as now, I embrace my vulnerability to relentless change, and how it feels—to, as they say, keep it all real.

Plus, the now-global merry-go-round of contagion is a strange way to awaken to the reality of interconnection. Looking deeper, it invites me to further embrace interbeing as the ground of my existence. That enables me to radically not know, within these times of great uncertainty.

And these three—nonself, impermanence, and interbeing—along with the related trio of curiosity, resilience, and not knowing—can't help but arouse my compassion, for myself and others. Along with any wisdom as such, compassion is always an appropriate response. (Coincidentally, sounding similar to the word "corona," the Sanskrit word for compassion is *karuna*.)

In and of itself, the nectar of compassion acts as a counterbalance to the preponderance these days of statistics and graphs, not to mention any toxic, downward-spiraling vortex of doom and gloom (our brain's negativity bias). Moreover, experiencing unsurpassable immeasurability allows heart and mind to expand as wide as need be.

Yet I cannot always maintain oceanic consciousness.[2] So, in considering the infinite light of love in endless life, I titrate it into particular colors of its spectrum.

> *may you be safe & secure, healthy & wholly well*
> *may you be truly happy*
> *may you touch peace know peace be peace teach peace*
> *may you thrive in a flourishing way*
> *may you remember your innate awakened nature*

If my words might be of any benefit, may the benefit be for all beings, and bring liberation. Stay well.

April 6, 2020

GARY GACH has been hosting Zen mindfulness fellowship weekly in San Francisco for a dozen years. Author, editor, and translator of nine books, and contributor to various anthologies and periodicals—more about him is available at GaryGach.com; social media at LinkTr.ee/GaryGach.

NOTES

1. After this text was composed, these words I've borrowed as epigraph "went viral." Some misattributed it to author Brené Brown, whose area of research has been courage, vulnerability, shame, and empathy. Sonya Renee Taylor is an author, poet, spoken word artist, speaker, humanitarian and social justice activist, educator, and founder of The Body Is Not an Apology movement (SonyaReneeTaylor.com).

2. "Because we cannot circle above all existence—sleepless, unbroken, boundless, glowing—we content ourselves with being submerged and awakening." —Martin Buber.

EXPOSED

Sherri Mitchell,
Weh'na Ha'mu Kwasset

PENOBSCOT NATION

I come from an Indigenous culture that has a rich storytelling tradition. These stories teach us how to interact with the places where we live; they help us to understand the changing circumstances of our lives; they provide us with a clear understanding of our place within creation, and they guide us toward a more harmonious way of being in relationship with the rest of life. In recent weeks, I have had the opportunity to contemplate the wisdom that our ancestors have maintained for us through these stories. I've marveled over their longevity, aware that the stories I grew up hearing were the same stories that my grandparents and great-grandparents had been told for generations before me. I've been awed by the incredible foresight and knowledge that the ancestors held and by the relevance of that wisdom to my contemporary life. As I've sat with the ancient wisdom of their words, I've realized that everything I need to know about living in this time was given to me by my ancestors generations ago.

Mathilda Sappier, a Wolastaq elder, began every story that she told with these words: "*kat yut atkuhkakon gin-te nit leyupon nita*" which means "this is not a story, it really happened." Her words have been replaying in my mind as I've watched these stories come to life around me. They are especially resonant when I think about the correlation between our current reality and our story of the first illness.

The Story of the First Illness

Long ago, during our first cycle of life, the two-legged (human beings), the youngest of all species, wandered away from the path of life. They had neglected their relationship with their relatives in the natural world and forgot their place within the sphere of creation. As a result, they lost their ability to speak the language of Nigwus Skiktomiq, *Mother Earth. They could no longer understand the words of the animals or hear the soft voices of the trees. Therefore, when the animals tried to warn them that they had departed from the path, their warnings went unheeded. When the trees tried to offer them guidance, their wisdom fell on deaf ears. The further the two-leggeds walked from the natural world, the further they traveled from the heart of their humanity. They stopped feeling the pain of Mother Earth and lost their compassion for their elders in the natural world—the trees, the rocks, and the waters. The two-legged began harming the body of Mother Earth and soon became a threat to the lives of other species, destroying their homes and eliminating their sources of food. After years of suffering the impacts of this destructive behavior, the animals called a council to determine what was to be done about the two-legged. They sat together for many days agonizing over their decision. Despite the actions of the two-legged, the animals loved them and continued to see them as lost children. They didn't want to harm them. However, they knew that something had to be done or the two-legged would eliminate the possibility of life for all living beings. Finally, they concluded that the two-legged must be taught that there were consequences for their destructive actions. They decided that they would give the two-legged illness to help them remember their connection to the web of life and to restore their compassion for their relatives in the natural world. The next time the two-legged took action that harmed the natural world, they received the illness that was sent to them by the animals. Since the two-legged had never seen illness before, it quickly spread, and they began to suffer and die.*

After watching the two-legged suffer, the plants began to feel sorry for them. So, they called a council to decide how they could help them. First, they recognized the wisdom of the animals and agreed that it was important for the two-legged to be taught a lesson, because of the risk they posed. Then, they crafted a solution that would help move the two-legged back onto the path of life. They decided that they would send a message to the two-legged in the form of a dream, and if one of them received this message and came to the animals with humility to ask for their guidance they would help them. The message was carried to the two-legged community and received by one of their elders. Upon waking, the elder told her family of the dream and then walked into the forest to ask for help. She humbly knelt before a beautiful tree and made an offering of tobacco and berries and asked for guidance with the illness that was plaguing her people. The next day, she went back into the forest and sat before a tiny plant, made an offering, and asked for the wisdom that the plant held. Every day, she returned to the forest and made her offerings to the plants and trees. After several days had passed, one of the plants spoke back to her and told her that they had seen the sincerity in her request. Then, they began to teach her the healing properties of the plants and told her which plants were needed to heal this illness. The grandmother remained humble and made an offering to each of the plants that carried the medicine she needed. Then, she carefully harvested a small amount from each plant, making sure that she did not take too much. She prepared the medicines according to the plants' instructions and gave it to those who were ill. Soon, they all became well and the community rejoiced. The people then pledged that they would never again wander away from the path of life. To seal that pledge they formed a sacred agreement, kci lakutawakon, *with the plants and animals. In that agreement, they promised that their children would forever hold the language of* Nigwus Skiktomiq, *and that they would always live in balance with their relatives in the natural world. And, so it was from that time forward that the two-legged lived in harmony with the world around them and their children held the language of Mother Earth in their mouths and their hearts. We,* Waponahkiyik, *are born of those who returned, and it is our responsibility to uphold their agreement.*

According to our teachings, this is the fourth cycle of life for human beings. Four times we have come here and four times we have fallen out of alignment with the natural order of life. We are now suffering the consequences of our collective actions. We have arrived at a crossroads where we must decide if we will continue walking the path of destruction that led us to this place, or if we will shift our direction and begin moving our lives back into harmony with the rest of creation.

In the very first story, which describes the creation of the universe, before Sky Woman came down from the stars and before the animals walked upon the Earth, *Kcinewisq* and *Kcimundu* were alone in the void. In this story, *Kcinewisq,* the sacred feminine, appears in the form of vibration and frequency, sound. *Kcimundu,* the sacred masculine, is a pool of shapeless matter that represents limitless potential. The story begins with *Kcinewisq* speaking into *Kcimundu.* As she speaks, the vibration and frequency of her words enter the pool that is *Kcimundu,* and the matter within him begins to organize and take form. She continues speaking until everything that is seen and unseen, known and unknown, within the universe has been created. Then, *Kcimundu* forms a protective shell around *Kcinewisq's* creation, encasing it in a single seed. This is the great seed of life. Once it has been formed, *Kcinewisq* begins to sing into the seed. First, she gently sings the creation song of each form that she created. Then she sings the song of life, a deep vibrational rhythm that rattles the seed and causes it to dance. The song builds slowly, and the seed expands and contracts with its quickening rhythm. This continues until the movement within the seed becomes strong enough to burst the shell and propel the life within across the universe.

This story is at the heart of our web of life teachings. It doesn't teach us that we are connected to the web of life. It teaches us that we are the web of life, one living being having simultaneous experiences of our self in multiple forms. We recognize that we are born from one body of matter. Therefore, we can never be separated. This understanding is best described in modern scientific terms as quantum entanglement. What quantum entanglement tells us is that any matter that was once connected physically can never be disconnected energetically. In our teachings, we recognize that we can never be disconnected energetically or spiritually.

In my book *Sacred Instructions,* I describe an experience that I had when I was a young girl. During this experience, the firm boundaries of my human body dissolved, and I merged with the larger body of the universe. While this was happening, my heart pulsed with the entire creation, and my breath rose and fell in rhythm with the world around me. In those fleeting moments, I realized that the person that I thought I was did not exist. I was not an individual expression living in relationship to other individual expressions. Instead, I was one living being learning to live in relationship with myself. This realization caused me to ask myself, "If I am part of one universal being, and am therefore present in every form that I encounter, how do I want to meet myself on the path?" Can I meet myself in all my myriad forms with curiosity and compassion, seeking true understanding? Am I capable of looking at an oppositional or harmful form and seeing my own reflection? Can I approach the aspects of myself that are out of alignment and dance them back into balance?

I've been asking myself these and similar questions for the past twenty-five years. Today, I'm asking some new questions. As I've searched for myself within the Coronavirus, I've seen a kaleidoscope of images that have led me back to our most ancient stories and some of our most lingering questions: Will we as a species make the changes necessary to move back into alignment with life, or will we continue following the path of destruction that leads to our extinction? Can we find our compassion for our relatives in the natural world and Mother Earth? Can we disengage our minds and our lives from the illusions of the material world and recognize that true wealth can only be measured through our support of one another? I believe we can, if we follow the guidance that is being given to us at this time.

The Coronavirus is providing us with a map for exploring our individual lives and our collective choices. By tracing the path that it offers, we can begin to understand the powerful lessons it has to teach us.

The first point on the map is exposure. This pandemic is exposing all the blind spots in our social lens. Many have claimed that this illness is the great equalizer; I disagree. There is no equity in access to shelter, water, food, or healthcare during this time. More than anything, this virus is highlighting the gross inequities and injustices within our societies. It's washing away the failing systems that we thought were foundational and showing us where our solid ground can truly be found.

In my book, I highlight four foundations of self-determined societies: food sovereignty, water sovereignty, energy sovereignty, and educational sovereignty. We need to build small collectives that manage these four foundational pillars within our local areas, to ensure more equity and to secure our basic needs when the larger systems fail, as they inevitably will. We also need to learn how to identify, grow, harvest, and process medicinal plants, so that we aren't left without health support when we are denied coverage by the for-profit health industry. When we allow our basic needs to be controlled by large profit-driven systems, we lose. One of the most important things that this moment is teaching us is to take responsibility for meeting our basic needs in more frugal and efficient ways. In other words, it's forcing us to grow up. Many people are realizing (some for the first time) that money does not come from trees, but oxygen does, and perhaps our next breath is more important than our next impulse buy.

As human activity has come to a near halt, NO_2 and CO_2 levels have dropped noticeably around the world, in some cases up to 30 percent. There is no irony in the fact that the virus attacking our respiratory systems is allowing Mother Earth to take her first deep breath in a century. There is only a powerful mirror, asking us to take a hard look at our impacts and showing us what's possible when we stop living lives of extreme excess.

After exposure comes incubation. As we collectively work to slow incubation of the virus by sheltering in place, we have an amazing opportunity to incubate our creative intelligence and deeper knowing. How we choose to occupy ourselves during this time of isolation is a predictor for how we will emerge. The things we focus on, the ways that we choose to entertain or occupy ourselves, the need that we have to distract ourselves, are all indicators of how we will surface from our shelters. If we can take advantage of this time and truly slow down our internal rhythms, let down the armor we have been required to don, and open ourselves up, we can incubate our individual creation songs[1] and our collective genius. The opportunity that we have to incubate our creative intelligence is filled with possibilities. This is a time for identifying and aligning with our deepest truths and bringing forward the dormant gifts that lie sleeping within us.

Once we discover the sparks of insight that live within our center, we must fan those sparks to flame. This is where the intense heat of fever is found on our Corona map. Here, we conduct a controlled burn of the debris that has covered our fertile ground. We burn off all the invasive plants (thoughts and ideas adopted from an outside source) and eliminate the local growths that don't belong there (family programming). A controlled burn can prevent a total burn-out; it can rejuvenate what is already there and protect the native habitat (your natural state of being). And, it encourages new growth.

As we move deeper into fever, we begin experiencing respiratory distress. On the psychospiritual level our lungs are the holders of our grief. Here, we deal with the pain of all that's been lost. What we've lost in the world—vital ecosystems, essential habitat, thousands of species, clean water.[2] Then, we must look at what has been lost within us—our connection to the source of life, our compassion for our relatives in the natural world, our relationship with Mother Earth, and our willingness to care for one another.

We must grieve the loss of friends and family members, those we are separated from while in isolation and those being taken from us permanently by the virus. And, finally, we must grieve our lost way of life, which will no longer serve us going forward.

This grieving process is the beginning of our letting go. I find it intriguing that a key component of letting go is to create physical distance from what you want to release. On a global scale, we have been positioned for this work. There is an incredibly powerful message in that. Now, we must decide what we are willing to release. This is where we confront death.

Knowing that death is coming may help to prepare us for the changes that it will bring, but it won't help alleviate the anxiety of anticipating its arrival. When we stand on death's door, we face the unknown. Fear of death is the most common fear held by human beings. Even when death is a blessed release, when it alleviates pain and suffering, we still hold on to our lives. However, if we look closely, we will realize that we have been shown the beauty and necessity of letting go since our first breath. The two things that are most essential to sustaining our lives, air and water, have shown us the danger of holding on too long and the relief that comes with letting go. We must take in both air and water in order to stay alive, but if we hold either indefinitely our lives are at risk. It is the process of taking in and then releasing that tells us we're alive. Where one breath ends, another begins. This informs us that death is a gateway to a new life. When we let go of what no longer serves us, we make space for the new to enter. An outgoing breath contains carbon dioxide and several other toxic gases that must be released from the body. If we attempted to retain those gases and bring them back into the body, it would very quickly become fatal. This is the lesson in this virus that is tied to our breath. It is telling us that we have to let go of the toxic breath that we've been forcing into the body of Mother Earth. It's telling us that we cannot go back to the way we were living before quarantine. It's forcing us into a position of letting go and showing us the collective power that we possess to alleviate the stress we are placing on our vital systems. In just over a month, the Coronavirus has shown us the consequences of our destruction of the natural world and the potential that we have to assist with the healing through organized, collective (in) action. This realization brings us to the final point on our map, rebirth.

> Every awakening is a rebirth. We are born and reborn repeatedly throughout our lives. We are born from the divine consciousness into our mother's womb. And, from our mother's womb we are born into the Earth. Then, we are born again and again, from within ourselves, breaking through layer after layer of illusion, until we are finally able to transcend those illusions and be reintegrated back into the divine consciousness. The time has passed for us to opt out of change. Change is upon us. The only question that remains is this: will we exit the planet, or alter our course?[3]

It's time for us to collectively exhale, to let go of the outdated systems and ideologies that are destroying our beloved Mother and our ability to sustain life. Now is the time to align our breath with the breath of Mother Earth, so we can move through this labor together and birth a new way of being into existence. This is the rebirth that our map is leading us toward. Where we go from here is up to us.

SHERRI MITCHELL (Weh'na Ha'mu Kwasset) was born and raised on the Penobscot Indian reservation. She received her juris doctorate and a certificate in Indigenous people's law and policy from the University of Arizona's James E. Rogers College of Law. Sherri is an alumna of the American Indian Ambassador program, and the Udall Native American Congressional Internship program. Sherri also received the Mahoney Dunn International Human Rights and Humanitarian Award, for research into human rights violations against Indigenous peoples. She was a longtime advisor to the American Indian Institute's Healing the Future Program and currently serves as an advisor to the Indigenous Elders and Medicine People's Council of North and South America. She is the founding director of the Land Peace Foundation, an organization dedicated to the global protection of Indigenous rights and the preservation of the Indigenous way of life. Prior to forming the Land Peace Foundation, Sherri served as a law clerk to the solicitor of the United States Department of Interior; as an associate with Fredericks, Peebles and Morgan Law Firm; a civil rights educator for the Maine Attorney General's Office; and as the staff attorney for the Native American Unit of Pine Tree Legal. Sherri is the author of the award-winning book *Sacred Instructions: Indigenous Wisdom for Living Spirit-Based Change.*

NOTES

1. Sherri Mitchell, "Creation Songs," chap. 1 in *Sacred Instructions: Indigenous Wisdom for Living Spirit-Based Change* (Berkeley: North Atlantic Books, 2018), 3–10.
2. Tony Greicius, ed., "Study: Third of Big Groundwater Basins in Distress," the website for NASA, June 16, 2015, https://www.nasa.gov/jpl/grace /study-third-of-big-groundwater-basins-in-distress.
3. Sherri Mitchell, "How We Got Here," chap. 4 in *Sacred Instructions: Indigenous Wisdom for Living Spirit-Based Change* (Berkeley: North Atlantic Books, 2018), 53–54.

MAKE THE BLEND, NOT WAR

Richard Strozzi-Heckler

As Covid-19 migrated from a bat body to a human body then accelerated to the global body, our historically conditioned tendencies predictably came to the foreground as our fatigued, out-of-date metaphors of war. "We're in a war," "This is combat," "The War Room," "We will destroy the enemy," "We're in a battle for our lives," "We need to be on the attack." This is a narrative of fear, the threat of the other, and our inability to deal with uncertainty, and it masks the opening that this pandemic offers. As shamans, curanderos, alternative medicine communities have voiced for millennia: It's not a disease, it's a healing crisis.

From this optic we could say that Covid-19 is not an enemy to war with but a guide who shares a web of interlocking, interdependent, ontological, and cellular relationships with us—an intelligent, powerful life force that is not only looking for a host in which it can photocopy its RNA but acting as a projection screen for our present state as a species and the conditions we've created on the planet.

King Covid, as I've heard it called in some neighborhoods, has heralded an initiatory moment for the evolution of our species and the planet. We have the opportunity to design a future different than the one that we've been blindly entering. Traditionally, initiations involve a struggle that overcomes an obstacle. It's a surrendering of the old and an embrace of the new. A romantic view perhaps, but a journey that exacts sweat, blood, and a rigorous look into the mirror.

In Aikido, a Japanese martial art, and in the somatic discourse (i.e., the healing, therapeutic, coaching, and embodiment arts that include bodywork, movement, breathwork, and the principles of Aikido), there's a central tenet and practice we call "making the blend." This means that when we're under some kind of threat, real or perceived, we take a moment to first center ourselves, noticing how we might be triggered and out of balance, and then we blend with, join with, the incoming energy. In Aikido it's using the energy of the attacker to neutralize his aggression, instead of neutralizing the person (read: go to war), bringing the confrontation into a harmonious reconciliation instead of a zero-sum game of winners and losers.

In the social context we can blend by embodying an open-hearted curiosity and authenticating the other's reality by trying to see their point of view. We may not agree with them, we may even be repulsed by them, but by opening ourselves and acknowledging the conditions that shaped their reality we also open the possibility of a future different than harm, cruelty, poisoning our water and air, dropping bombs. Some might call this compassionate wisdom.

What I'm suggesting is that using the metaphors of war in this pandemic is also infectious. Stories infect our nervous system; narratives infect our spirits. The metaphorical virus of violence may be what brought us here in the first place. When we take the shape of aggression and violence we are predisposed to fear, anxiety, and panic. To make the blend doesn't mean we don't heal and cure and find a solution for ourselves; it doesn't mean we capitulate or give up our position; it doesn't mean we can't fight for what we care about. It means we recognize our interconnectedness with life and choose a path that is an affirmation of life. We're able to see past our deeply conditioned strategies for survival, to see beyond our lifetime and into the future of our children and grandchildren.

Try it for a moment: Take the shape of fighting, of destroying the opponent. Fists clenched to hit; jaw set to oppress; crouch and round the shoulders. To be less of a target, narrow the eyes, extending the head forward of the chest; the breath is high and short. Now take the shape of making the blend, of listening to the life energy that flows through all of us. You're upright in harmony with the downward pull of gravity; your hands are alive and relaxed for optimum choice of action; your eyes are relaxed, you have a panoramic vision; your legs and feet are connecting you to the ground; your breath is low and rhythmic.

This is something we can practice. It's a choice we can make.

Making a blend with King Covid at a molecular, cellular, interpersonal, social, and ecological level is asking us to see our co-dependence with it; to reflect on how we are projecting our profound panic on this virulent form of life, and how we have invited it in. Richard Preston, a scientific writer of fiction, non-fiction, and screenplays who has studied viruses and epidemics for decades, traces how viruses often emerge from the degradation of ecosystems, particularly savannas and tropical rainforests. He explains how viruses in a damaged ecosystem tend to mutate and adapt quickly, noting that "viruses leaving a non-human host crash into a human host like rats leaving a ship." Since we are the authors of our environmental crisis, can we own that perhaps we actually invited the virus into our midst; can we see that the genocide of Indigenous people is a virus; that our fear is a virus? Now we are being asked straight up to examine the consumer chaos of late-stage capitalism, the economic hardship of the poor, the racial divide, the social inequity. These are questions of leadership. The mirror of King Covid reflects that our current leadership is infected with a virus of aggression and fear: brittle, self-serving, contracted.

From the perspective of the blend, the metaphors and narratives of war are limiting, if not harmful. If we choose to act from the bigger picture, then we must blend with what King Covid is guiding us to. But don't get me wrong: Blending also means giving our heartfelt gratitude and help to the first responders and healthcare workers; extending our compassion and help to those who are ill, to those who have lost loved ones; assisting those who are experiencing severe economic hardships; and respecting social distancing, washing our hands, and observing sheltering as civic duty as well as an extended moment of spiritual refuge.

Let's make the blend and not war.

TAKE IT EASY, BUT TAKE IT

RICHARD

RICHARD STROZZI-HECKLER is a 7th dan shihan in Aikido and has a Ph.D. in Psychology. He is author of eight books including *In Search of the Warrior Spirit, The Art of Somatic Coaching,* and *The Leadership Dojo.* He is the founder of Strozzi Institute, the Center for Leadership and Mastery. From 2002 to 2007, he was an advisor to NATO and the Supreme Allied Commander of Europe General Jim Jones, formally the national security advisor under President Obama.

MEDICAL INFORMATION
AND HEALING MODALITIES

MEDICAL INFORMATION AND HEALING MODALITIES

Meryl Nass

This paper is designed to help readers understand the new coronavirus and why it has inevitably led to the quarantine measures currently imposed. I will refer to the virus as the COVID-19 virus, as does the WHO, instead of using the official but confusing name SARS-CoV-2. The official name of the disease is COVID-19.

HISTORICAL BACKGROUND

A novel coronavirus, similar to the virus that caused the 2003 SARS (severe acute respiratory syndrome) epidemic, appeared in China in December 2019 or earlier. It caused a new syndrome with primarily respiratory symptoms. The degree of rapid spread was phenomenal in the megacity of Wuhan, population 11 million. Wuhan ran out of gear, doctors, hospital beds. The Chinese government was able to commandeer supplies, doctors, and nurses from other provinces, and retrain medical professionals to cope with an extraordinarily infectious, and sometimes lethal, virus.[1] This included having doctors put on full PPE—being covered head to toe, and not changing out the gear for a full twelve-hour shift. No bathroom breaks, no meals. They have worked seven days a week, with no time off. Doctors have been housed in hotels and unable to visit family members—not that they wanted to visit, since contact might spread the disease to their families. With extraordinary lockdowns, China gained control of its epidemic. The Western press portrayed this as another example of China's authoritarian regime. Little did they know.

The Chinese report that almost all people who catch this disease are symptomatic. But 80–85 percent have only mild symptoms and can be left to care for themselves at home with rest and fluids. However, about 15 percent of those diagnosed required hospitalization, due to lack of oxygen from extensive viral pneumonia. One third of these, or 5 percent of all cases, required ICU care and frequently needed to be placed on mechanical ventilation. Some percentage of total cases, probably about 2–4 percent in China but about 8–10 percent in Italy, which has an older population, could not be saved despite the most aggressive medical measures and died of this disease. Italy found that considerably more of its population required ICU care.[2]

It is possible that many more people than we know have asymptomatic cases and that our statistics make things look worse than they are. I certainly hope so. But I have seen no evidence to support this hope.

I had assumed the Chinese, who were practiced in handling such diseases after SARS, would get this one under control expeditiously, and much more quickly than has happened.

This assumption turned out to be wrong. Why? Apparently, while this virus's mortality rate is not as high as mortality from the SARS (10 percent) or MERS virus (33 percent mortality), it has other features that make it *much more contagious*. These were not immediately appreciated in China, and it took far too long for this to be appreciated elsewhere in the world.

THE COVID-19 VIRUS IS EXTRAORDINARILY CONTAGIOUS[3]

1. The COVID-19 virus led to 1,000 times as much virus (500,000,000 viral particles on a swab)[4] present in the throat compared to the SARS

virus (500,000 particles). While we don't yet know how many viral particles it takes to cause an infection, if there are 1,000 times as many particles being expelled with a cough or sneeze, or when simply breathing, breathing indoor air shared with someone who is infected is likely to be a significant risk factor.

2. Unlike most infections, this virus appears to be contagious even before symptoms occur and after patients appear to have resolved the infection.[5] SARS was contagious only after several days of illness, enabling effective quarantines to be implemented. For this virus, the highest viral titers are measured at the beginning of illness, prior to diagnosis. When the COVID-19 virus is contagious when cases are asymptomatic, there is no way to impose effective quarantines on the infected without testing everyone.

On average, it takes five days from exposure until onset of symptoms,[6] but may take up to fourteen days and rarely longer.

INADEQUATE TESTING

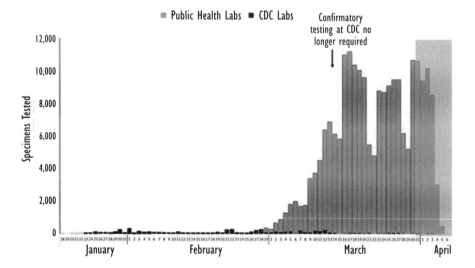

The CDC restricted testing to all but a tiny number of those with compatible symptoms, as the CDC acknowledges in its graph, above. Had there been the availability of widespread reverse transcriptase PCR testing, or had other types of tests been made available, and if the US had been able to test cases with minimal or no symptoms, maybe the US or other nations could have instituted quarantines that stopped spread. But as you know, the CDC made the inexplicable decision to restrict US testing by allowing only the test CDC had developed to be used,[7] a test that was both unnecessarily cumbersome and faulty,[8] and to test only those who almost certainly were infected. This slowed down the development of better and more accessible tests by private, university, and state public health labs. CDC's ban on other tests was only lifted on February 28. (Tom Frieden, former CDC Director, has called for an independent panel to investigate what went wrong.)[9]

After Feb. 28, the FDA offered to approve new COVID virus tests using its authority under an Emergency Use Authorization. But that, too, held up the use of new tests until the FDA approved them. Finally, to avoid another bottleneck, the FDA allowed any entity to start using its own tests and apply for approval later.

THE PROLONGED DURATION OF INFECTIVITY

One study found that the *median length of time during which patients were contagious was twenty days*. One patient had detectable virus for thirty-seven days. The duration of contagion might even extend further in some cases, because patients who died tended to remain contagious throughout their course. Let me repeat myself: Patients were contagious before they showed symptoms, during their symptomatic phase, and even after they recovered. This makes it impossible to identify those who are spreading the disease. It also makes it impossible to keep hospitals (and other indoor spaces) clean.

AIRBORNE VS. DROPLET SPREAD

When you cough or breathe, particles of air, virus, and water are expelled. The old dogma held that most illnesses produce exhaled particles greater than 5µ in size (droplets), which fall to the ground within 3 feet of the person producing them. Particles smaller than 5µ in size could travel further, up to 6 feet away from the person who expelled them. However, very small particles could stay suspended in air for hours or days. Newer research tells us that we breathe out particles of many different sizes,[10] and that 3' and 6' distancing does not account for airborne particles. Some of what we exhale falls close to us, while other particles remain suspended in the air for indefinite periods and can travel on air currents.

Once particles fall out of the air, they usually contain viable virus and contaminate the surfaces onto which they fall. The COVID virus is more dangerous as a large droplet but can still spread as tiny particles that remain suspended in air for hours and perhaps a few days.[11] Indoor air becomes a risk, especially in closed spaces like elevators, which are used by large numbers of people.

Negative-pressure rooms in hospitals suck indoor air out of infected patients' rooms, preventing virus from contaminating hospital halls and other areas. But there are not enough negative-pressure rooms for COVID-19 patients, especially in ICUs and ERs. So you cannot keep the air and surfaces in a hospital entirely free of virus. ICUs with all their equipment will be contaminated. The only thing to do is to have everyone working in the hospital wear full airborne personal protective equipment, from head to toe, all day long. This is what Chinese doctors had to do. But what will happen to the other, non-COVID patients? Some will be exposed. Visitors must be banned. This is probably why hospitals try to empty themselves of patients—both for the predicted onslaught of new patients and to minimize the number of patients who will be exposed to the COVID-19 virus while being treated for something else.

One solution is to create separate hospital facilities for COVID patients and for everybody else. This, of course, requires being able to test and identify those with infection.

DURATION OF INFECTIVITY ON SURFACES

Bacteria and viruses don't die like people do. People are either alive or dead. But the COVID virus, like other microorganisms, is found in colonies or groups and their number slowly falls over time. The number of viruses in these groups "decays" logarithmically, instead of dying all at once.

Let's say you have 1 million viral particles on a copper surface. Copper, by the way, is the surface that destroys virus the fastest. After one half-life, which usually is, say, one hour, half will still be viable: 500,000. After another hour, half of those, or 250,000, will remain viable. After 24 hours, you will no longer have viable viral particles. Virus lives longer on glass, plexiglass, and steel surfaces. This applies to *uncleaned* surfaces.

So, if you don't handle contaminated items for several days, probably enough of the virus will have died to make your risk negligible. But if you want to touch something sooner, you will need to decontaminate the surface. G. Kampf, D. Todt, S. Pfaender, and E. Steinmann, in their article "Persistence of coronaviruses on inanimate surfaces and their inactivation with biocidal agents," present good answers for what works and how long you need to keep your disinfectant in contact with the surface.[12] I summarize:

> **Bleach (sodium hypochlorite) 0.21% dilution on a surface for one minute.** Different bottles of bleach have different concentrations, so calculate your dilution accordingly. One part hypochlorite per thousand parts water. Roughly ⅓–½ cup bleach per gallon water.
> **Hydrogen peroxide 0.5% dilution for one minute.**
> **Alcohol 70% or more concentration, for 30 seconds.** Lower concentrations may also work but testing was limited.

Be aware that virus lives on cardboard, paper, clothing for days. Washing clothes daily, not wearing outdoor shoes into the house, and frequent showering will all reduce the amount of virus you harbor.

PERSONAL PROTECTIVE EQUIPMENT (PPE) FOR HEALTHCARE WORKERS

What is full airborne personal protective equipment? This is what healthcare workers used for the Ebola epidemic. We use a little less gear for active tuberculosis. It means being covered head to toe with disposable suits, caps, gloves, shoe covers, nose/mouth and eye coverage, and often a clear visor in front of the face.

I have rarely had to use eye protection with patients before, nor was it considered necessary to use a plexiglass face shield. But the diseases that hospital doctors were previously exposed to (apart from Ebola) were treatable, and we almost never got them, and virtually never died from them if we did. This disease is different.

An estimated 1,700 healthcare workers (HCWs) in Italy became infected (8 percent of the total number of cases) only a month after the country identified its first case. A number of healthcare workers globally have died from the disease.

THE SYMPTOMS OF COVID-19

The most common early symptoms of this infection, in roughly descending order, are fever, fatigue, dry cough, headaches, loss of appetite, shortness of breath, muscle pain, occasional sputum production. There is usually no runny nose, diarrhea, or vomiting, but they occasionally occur.

The severe syndrome (based partly on unpublished emails from doctors in the field):

A normal respiratory virus may temporarily fill your lungs with inflammatory materials, but most people, even with severe disease, can be kept alive for a week or two and their body will fight off the infection. As long as you keep them oxygenated they recover. Of course, those with severe underlying conditions may succumb to a final hit by the virus.

This viral disease is different.

1. It lasts longer: People with severe disease tend to spend 2–6 weeks in the hospital, much longer than normal. That means they take up many more hospital beds, and contaminate hospitals longer.

2. It causes a relatively mild viral illness, which usually includes a viral pneumonia, for about a week, then patients may suddenly "crash" with respiratory failure. Acute Respiratory Distress Syndrome (ARDS), which has a mortality around 30–40 percent, is a common complication. Cytokine storm is another COVID-19 complication, which has a high mortality rate and may be part of the ARDS syndrome. Those who survive may have significant scarring of their lungs and face a prolonged recuperation.

3. It can affect multiple organs. Some patients have died of cardiac failure (myocarditis) after seeming to start recovering from the viral pneumonia. Virus has been found in heart muscle, gut, and liver. It has been isolated from urine and stool, although a minority of patients develop nausea, vomiting, or diarrhea. Some patients develop shock and/or multiorgan failure.

While a higher percentage of the elderly and infirm are dying from COVID-19, there are plenty of fit young people being stricken with severe illness or death. Doctors have no idea why some healthy people develop severe disease and others don't. Probably this is due to genetic differences that have yet to be identified. No adult is in a completely safe demographic.

The period during which testing and isolation of cases would have halted spread is over. That window was missed. That opportunity is gone.

The term "flattening the curve" means slowing down spread of virus, even though (presumably) the same number of people will be infected by the end of the epidemic. It means that the epidemic will be slowed, and last longer, but large numbers of unnecessary deaths caused by a crash of the healthcare system will be avoided. And that is huge. It also buys time to manufacture the masks, ventilators, and drugs that will be needed. It buys time to find new drugs that may be effective.

Isolation from everyone but the people you live with is critical. Please take this situation seriously, and do your best to comply. My recommendations on how best to avoid infection are posted on this website:

https://anthraxvaccine.blogspot.com/2020/03
/protecting-yourself-from-covid-19-nass.html

Meryl Nass, M.D., is an internal medicine physician who did groundbreaking work analyzing the world's largest anthrax epidemic and showing it was due to biological warfare. She has investigated the Cuban neuropathy epidemic for the Cuban Ministry of Health, helped the World Bank respond to the anthrax letters, and advised the director of national intelligence on domestic biological terrorism. She has written on the anthrax letters case and West Africa's Ebola epidemic and provided testimony to six different Congressional committees. Her current work includes treating tick-borne diseases and studying vaccine safety in addition to understanding and ameliorating the COVID-19 pandemic.

1. Yuexuan Chen, "A Wuhan Doctor on the Front Lines: 'Fear to the First Degree,'" *Medscape,* March 11, 2020, https://www.medscape.com/viewarticle/926598.

2. Mary Van Beusekom, "Doctors: COVID-19 pushing Italian ICUs toward collapse," *CIDRAP,* March 16, 2020, https://www.cidrap.umn.edu/news-perspective/2020/03/doctors-covid-19-pushing-italian-icus-toward-collapse.

3. Mary Van Beusekom, "Study highlights ease of spread of COVID-19 viruses," *CIDRAP,* March 09, 2020, https://www.cidrap.umn.edu/news-perspective/2020/03/study-highlights-ease-spread-covid-19-viruses.

4. Roman Wölfel, Victor M. Corman, Wolfgang Guggemos et al., "Virological assessment of hospitalized cases of coronavirus disease 2019," Preprint, submitted March 8, 2020, https://www.medrxiv.org/content/10.1101/2020.03.05.20030502v1.full.pdf.

5. Helen Branswell, "We're learning a lot about the coronavirus. It will help us assess risk," *STAT,* March 6, 2020, https://www.statnews.com/2020/03/06/were-learning-a-lot-about-the-coronavirus-it-will-help-us-assess-risk/

6. Van Beusekom, "Ease of spread."

7. Peter Whoriskey and Neena Satija, "How U.S. coronavirus testing stalled: Flawed tests, red tape and resistance to using the millions of tests produced by the WHO," *Washington Post,* March 16, 2020, https://www.washingtonpost.com/business/2020/03/16/cdc-who-coronavirus-tests.

8. Carolyn Y. Johnson, Laurie McGinley, and Lena H. Sun, "A faulty CDC coronavirus test delays monitoring of disease's spread," *Washington Post,* Febuary 25, 2020, https://www.washingtonpost.com/health/2020/02/25/cdc-coronavirus-test/.

9. Whoriskey and Satija, "U.S. coronavirus testing stalled."

10. James Atkinson et al., eds., *Natural Ventilation for Infection Control in Health-Care Settings,* (Geneva: World Health Organization, 2009), https://www.ncbi.nlm.nih.gov/books/NBK143281/.

11. Sharon Begley, "The new coronavirus can likely remain airborne for some time. That doesn't mean we're doomed," *STAT,* March 16, 2020, https://www.statnews.com/2020/03/16/coronavirus-can-become-aerosol-doesnt-mean-doomed.

12. G. Kampf, D. Todt, S. Pfaender, and E. Steinmann, "Persistence of coronaviruses on inanimate surfaces and their inactivation with biocidal agents," *Journal of Hospital Infection* 104 (2020): 246–51, https://www.journalofhospitalinfection.com/article/S0195-6701(20)30046-3/pdf.

CORONAVIRUS (COVID-19)

Herbal and Holistic Perspectives

Matthew Wood

A note from the author: It is now clear, if it wasn't before, that every case is different, that there are different herbs in every household, and different skills. Use what you can: hot water drinks if nothing else, and cooling water if that is what you crave. Do what feels right for each person. Don't believe "the experts," including this paper: Observe carefully with your own senses and form your own judgments.

The emphasis in this approach to the coronavirus is on the *symptoms* and their interpretation and possible treatment from a holistic standpoint. That includes energetic indicators (hot, cold, damp, dry, tense, relaxed) and organ-specificity, since so many organs and tissues are involved. The need for "sophisticated, organ-specific treatment" is also commented on by prominent herbal writer Stephen Harrod Buhner.[1] I highly recommend his June 2020 paper on the subject.

In traditional herbalism, which I have practiced for more than 35 years, the emphasis is placed on strengthening the body to remove or disrupt the environment in which the organism likes to make its home—or at least to match the symptoms with a remedy. In a case like this it would be nice to be able to kill the virus, but so far that seems to elude us. The holistic approach was put very nicely by A. Bruce Boraas, a longtime Minnesota practitioner of natural medicine:[2]

> The better the circulation, the better the elimination. The better the elimination, the better the interior. The better the metabolism, the better the breakdown of waste products.

This is the approach of our medical ancestors: the holistic, naturopathic, herbal, granny, and traditional healers of the world. Unlike a purely scientific writer, I have also used the "anecdotal approach," letting people tell their stories in their own words.

I have been reporting on the symptoms of coronavirus from the holistic or energetic perspective since January 26, 2020. I have been modifying information based on increased data and understanding. I started with the emphasis on the pulmonary symptoms because that is what came through in the first reports out of China. However, it was soon clear that the virus was actively attacking the heart as well as the lungs. It was suspected—and then confirmed—that it sometimes presented as a gastrointestinal condition. Then the nervous system was shown to be involved—loss of sense of smell and taste and inflammation of the eyes. The liver and kidneys are naturally exhausted keeping up with the waste products of any disease, but especially one that moves so rapidly—so they too were implicated. The brain was shown to be involved in yet more cases. What seemed at first to be largely a disease of older, impaired populations was also found to attack young, healthy people. In May 2020 it was recognized that blood coagulation is an important factor.

Evidence has accrued that the virus is mutating rapidly. As a result, my viewpoint has morphed and changed again and again, and I now offer the following advice: Each case, each person, is different, and individuals must figure out for themselves the most appropriate remediation. Holism says there are many potential treatments—not necessarily for killing the virus but for strengthening the body's response at each turn, so that one is not overwhelmed by the disease.

The first detailed paper from Chinese herbal/acupuncturist practitioners in China that I received was "Diagnosis and Treatment of Pneumonitis with a New Coronavirus Infection," provided by Mayway Herbs, translated and forwarded to me by Jen Ciccolella.[3] To this I added information from "Report from the Front Line in Wuhan" by Liu Lihong, Institute for the Research and Preservation of Classical Chinese Medicine, Guanxi University of Traditional Chinese Medicine (TCM).[4] Then we had pictures of tongues and a good roundup of symptoms from John K. Chen, Ph.D., Pharm.D., O.M.D., L.Ac., "Medical Records from a Young and Brave Female Traditional Chinese Medicine (TCM) Doctor on Fighting the COVID-19, Part III."[5]

Western doctors are not as symptom-conscious as their Oriental counterparts, but I found that the observations of an anonymous "ER MD in New Orleans" gave a useful timeline and symptom pictures.[6]

The herbalist I know with the most direct experience of respiratory problems in a COVID-laced area is Judith Lieblein of Marin County, California. Before I had direct personal experience I relied upon her clinical perspectives.[7]

THE MECHANISM OF COVID INFECTION

Coronavirus enters the body through the ACE2 receptors in the membranes of the surfactant cells in the alveoli of the lungs. The alveoli are little terminal air sacs at the end of the bronchial tree. They exchange water and CO_2 from inside the lungs for oxygen from outside the body. Surfactant cells help to keep the alveolar surfaces from sticking together so that they open easily with each respiration. The ACE2 receptors, when stimulated, push up the blood pressure. This would explain why so many people feel a weight on their chest as the blood pressure increases, and why high blood pressure is a risk factor. Damage to surfactant cells would make it harder for the alveoli to open with each breath. The immune system responds to stimulate fibroblasts to repair the thin membrane of the surfactant cells. This leads to an over-production by the fibroblasts, resulting in fibrosis or scar tissue. This is why the ventilators are used to push gases back and forth across this membrane.

Cytokines are a necessary part of the immune process. They are stimulated by the arachidonic acid or inflammatory cascade, i.e., by fever. As waste products build up and more and more organs are engaged and the viral load is high, the cytokines can overproduce, causing the famous "storm." The ER doctor mentioned above commented, "You can literally watch it happen in a matter of hours," finishing the case.

Blockage of the alveoli and fluids backs up water and blood in the pleural lining around the lungs and in the lungs themselves and, as widely reported on the internet, people are literally drowning in their own blood and fluids.

In late April a new factor was discovered. About 20–30 percent of the critically ill develop blood clots that can be deadly. The origin of these clots is not known as I write. Young people, who normally don't get strokes, are dying from them. Extensive clotting may explain low oxygen levels in the blood.[8] Blood-thinners are now being used with apparent success to assist these patients.[9] The full implications are not yet known. "Placentas in COVID-positive pregnant women show injury with blood circulation and clotting," said a headline in the *Chicago Tribune* (May 22, 2020).[10]

Although the virus usually enters through the lungs, in other cases the primary effect is through the ACE2 receptors in the GI tract. This causes gastric or intestinal symptoms. Some people have both respiratory and GI involvement. In addition to the other pressures on the lungs, spasm in the stomach would translate to the diaphragm, interfering with breathing. Hold your diaphragm still, readers, and see if you can breathe! The diaphragm may also weaken.

The liver is also affected. Initial statistics from China suggest that symptoms of liver damage are higher in those who die compared to those who live.[11] This same source also reports that bile duct epithelium and hepatocytes have ACE2 receptor sites, so they too may be attacked by COVID. These receptors are more numerous in the bile ducts and are "known to play important roles in liver regeneration and immune response," according to the article. There was also evidence of drug-induced liver damage from antibiotics, steroids, and antivirals. The New Orleans ER doctor comments: "Do not use steroids, it makes this worse. Push out to your urgent cares to stop their usual practice of steroid shots for their URI/bronchitis."[12] When the liver can't process hormones and neurotransmitters correctly, multiple systems can become disordered.

The brain and neurological system seem to be involved: The organs of smell and taste are often knocked off line, the eyes may be inflamed, there may be a sense of oppressive fullness or even burning in the head, and outright hallucinations of the dead are possible—as newsman Chris Cuomo reported on his own case.[13]

A characteristic found in people with a spiritual orientation is *meaningful visions* and *dreams,* including information about COVID or remedies to use in the pandemic. "Weird dreams" are attested to by many, according to a *National Geographic* article.[14] However, this article attributes the symptom to the boredom induced by quarantine. I think this is a ridiculous grasp at a simplistic explanation for something far more complex. We have dream centers in the brain; there is no reason why COVID cannot act directly upon them. The lockdown was not a consideration in Chris Cuomo's case since he had only been in quarantine for a day or two when he had a hallucination.

Blood tests show that initially immune cells are low; the immune system is suppressed by COVID.

CAN HERBS HELP?

Of all the cases sent to me by correspondents, my favorite was sent early in the epidemic from Italy.[15] This case illustrates the importance of hot remedies throughout, *in some presentations.* Notice the severe aggravation from a cooling food. A heroic wife writes:

Case History, Efeturi: *Covid Italia. The symptoms began but were not noticed for a few days. I noticed on the 19th March the tips of his hands were becoming blue like there was no blood flow to that part. Slight fever (I didn't measure it) but he felt mildly hot on touch. But the most challenging symptom was difficulty breathing— which took him to the ER. Chest congestion; he progressed from lying down and feeling relief to lying down and feeling no relief at all. Talking was a struggle. He says the pain made him angry to even talk to me.*

Treatment: General Strategy throughout: I made the room constantly hot and got an extra electric heater, which was turned to his chest region. And he was lying under an electric blanket. Substituted teas for drinking water where I put 3 bags of cinnamon tea, green tea, and Indian black tea together. Changed clothes and beddings every day and gave hot baths. I didn't practice isolation (we slept in same bed, I was constantly with him) but ensured daily we both changed clothing and I also took everything I gave him in smaller quantities. Sanitized my hands and door handles, bathroom after every bath.

Day 1. I had just a few items around me like onions and garlic so I started him on a fresh garlic clove. He felt relief after about 4 minutes after eating (I counted this) but the pain and congestion came back within 30 minutes. I thought to add something more so I made garlic, ginger, and strawberry finely cut in honey (he didn't like and only took this on the first day so I don't think this worked for him). Had to rush him to the ER because he could not breathe, was very anxious and panicking. He spent all day there and all tests were conducted and a potential diagnosis of COVID-19 was made and a lung xray showed an inflamed bronchi. At the end of the day, ER said nothing could be done and he was asked to go home and stay indoors, isolating self for 14 days and call a particular number if the chest congestion continued the next day. An official diagnosis of "cough and chest congestion" was made. COVID-19 test was done and the result was not given to him but was to be communicated to him later the next day. Tested positive.

He was never coughing and did not cough at all except during steam sessions. We knew he had the virus because over the next days the chest congestion continued, but we didn't call the number because we wanted to try with garlic for one week to see if it goes away and if not then we call the emergency number. Meals were soups and green veggie broths with a lot of hot spices and chili peppers (can't remember the exact spice ingredient in the hot spice mix as I got them ground from a friend a long time ago). I gradually increased the garlic and added in practically everything. These episodes usually began during the evenings and lasted up until 3 am before falling asleep. Within this time I am either giving him hot teas to drink, massages with tea extract, and more garlic. Teas and steam coverings with garlic, ginger, onions and garlic peels, citrus peels induced sweating, and after this a hot bath followed by more tea and garlic.

Day 8. Yesterday he sat in the sun for 2 hours (not directly in the sun but just by the window) and he felt so much better with no symptoms and was so excited. This is the 8th day and he feels so much better, but noticed slight breathing difficulty and slight pain at the lower sides of the ribs. Just got mullein tea today. He drank the first cup and I want to continue with this plus the garlic. I noticed after teas etc he had frequent bowel movements and urination and lots of white sputum.

I want to emphasize that simple kitchen herbs can potentially save lives. **Garlic** brings down blood pressure by catalyzing nitric oxide, which is released by the blood vessels for this purpose. It has a temporary, daily effect rather than a long-term cure, but that is what we need in an acute disease. Also it may be good for hypoxia (lack of oxygen to the body tissues). Peter Jackson-Main, NIMH, herbal teacher at a naturopathic college in London, notes that "the Sherpas in Nepal apparently use garlic to enable oxygen absorption at high altitude."[16]

VITAMINS AND MINERALS

Vitamin D3. From the first whispers of the pandemic, holistic practitioners were suggesting supplementation with this vitamin. In addition to its more famous application in building bones with calcium, it has a proven track record in reducing influenza and the old coronavirus infections. A 2008 landmark article, "On the epidemiology of influenza," in *Virology Journal* began with the fact that vitamin D3 is a necessary component in the health of the innate immune system.[17] Since it is produced in human beings through sunlight hitting the skin, this also explains why influenza is seasonal, explosive, coincidental in countries of similar latitude, spreads rapidly, then disappears. Vitamin D is the most researched and important supplement for COVID-19 in this paper.

    Zinc. This trace element possesses numerous essential functions in the body. A review article entitled "The Role of Zinc in Antiviral Immunity" states: "An abundance of evidence has accumulated over the past 50 y[ears] to demonstrate the antiviral activity of zinc against a variety of viruses, and via numerous mechanisms."[18] It is, therefore, being recommended for COVID. Furthermore, there is evidence that zinc works synergistically with chloroquine/hydroxyquine, a drug suggested as a treatment for the virus. The combination gets zinc inside cells to assist in antiviral enzyme activities.[19]

    Vitamin C. Another basic remedy here, which is gathering more and more support, is Vitamin C. Ascorbic acid strengthens the endothelium (base layer of the mucosa lining, which viruses attack) and is also a circulatory catalyst. The full vitamin C "package" not only contains ascorbic acid but vitamins P and K, which thin the blood.

HOMEOPATHIC REMEDIES

Dana Ullman, a well-known, experienced practitioner and writer on homeopathy, states, "There is NO remedy that fits all, though the most common ones are Arsenicum, Bryonia, Gelsemium, Camphora, Phosphorus, Lycopodium, Antimonium tart . . . for starters."[20]

Arsenicum album 30x, 30c (**homeopathic Arsenic**). This has been recommended as a specific by the government of India.[21] It is especially for anguish, anxiety, and fear. It also matches the symptoms of aggravation at night, anxiety at night, and it is reliable in many acute microbial presentations; also in chronic and constitutional cases.

Cinchona officinalis, China officinalis (**homeopathic Quinine**). Many people familiar with homeopathy have taken this remedy due to the reports about chloroquine or hydroxychloroquine, a synthetic derivative from this long-recognized malarial medicinal plant.

FLOWER ESSENCES

Julia Graves, an experienced herbalist and flower essence practitioner in Germany, writes: "Flower essences as vibrational or energy medicine do not kill viruses. However, we all know that the more we feel happy, loving and vibrant, the less likely we are to catch what is going around." She recommends Yellow Daylily (light-heartedness), Lily of the Valley ("no love in the world"), Hellebore (fear), Spear Thistle ("spiritual warrior"), Grape Hyacinth (weakness of voice and chest).[22]

I recommend the Bach flower essence Holly (more about that to come). My friend Wendy Fogg, of Misty Meadows Herbal Center in Durham, New Hampshire, recommends Borage (emotional exhaustion) and Wild Rose (fear). We agreed that Holly would combine well with these.[23]

MEDICAL DEVICES

The importance of having a pulse oximeter to monitor oxygen levels in the blood will become apparent in this article.

PREPARATION/PREVENTION

There is no proof that prevention of COVID is possible except through social distancing measures that are being practiced throughout the world. However, we can strengthen ourselves in advance. The use of vitamin D3, as described above, has been proven to be strongly preventative in influenza and the previous coronaviruses. Other preventative measures include the following.

Rest and Hydration. The simple practices for avoiding complications from influenza and ordinary (pre-COVID-19) coronavirus remain in effect.[24] Warm water has been recommended by doctors in India, Italy, and Spain, since flu and COVID often begin with chills. A cold drink contributed to a relapse in my own case.

Protect the Mucosal Lining. The "front line" of the immune system is the "intrinsic epithelial barrier," in other words, the mucosal and dermal lining of the body. N-acetylcholine is the substance from which cell membranes are made; it is contained in lecithin and eggs or can be supplemented directly. In a quick search I gathered information on strengthening the epithelium of the intestines from an article published in China.[25] Positive agents include fatty acids, especially linoleic acid and oleanolic acid, fruits including citrus, several rosaceae (raspberry, apple, strawberries), herbs including Citrus peel, Astragalus, Sage (Chinese, probably also Western), Magnolia officinalis, Moringa, Coptis (similar to Goldenseal), Mango butter, and other substances.

The layer under the epithelium should also be strengthened—this would be the **mesothelium** or connective-tissue layer. The polymers of this layer provide the "tight junctions" between the cells and need to be healthy. Immune functions are also found in the mesothelium. This layer is strengthened by mucilages, and the junctions can be tightened by flavonoids (Rose family, for instance). Recommended mucilages include Marshmallow Root, Fenugreek Seed (especially because it is also warming and contains fatty acids), Opuntia, Aloe Vera, and Gotu Kola. Horsetail, though not mucilaginous, is excellent for strengthening the connective tissue.

The **endothelium** is the layer beneath the epi- and mesothelium; it has been shown to be strengthened by Vitamin C.[26]

The **thermoregulatory system** opens and closes the pores of the skin, mucosa, and internal serous membranes. This is the basis of old-time and herbal medicine. The theory is: warm the center, thin the fluids, keep the pores open to discharge healthy secretions onto the epithelial surface. Warming, thinning/expectorating, and opening remedies include Lomatium, Angelica, Fenugreek, Elecampane, Hyssop, various mints, and others.[27]

The importance of prevention and taking a serious attitude toward COVID is highlighted in this cautionary tale from Canadian herbalist Christine Dennis (mentioned under Encephalopathy):

> I underestimated this virus. It is an angry little virus. I was not taking my preventative herbs and that was the first big misstep on my part. I was saving them for those that are more vulnerable than I. I was also late to start my herbs once it hit because I again wanted to save them. Misstep number 2. Then I was getting on top of it with saunas but got feeling like I was getting on top of it and stopped the saunas. Misstep number 3. Then I thought I was over the hump and eased off on what all I was doing, so that was when I got hit with a second round of it. Misstep number 4.

STAGES AND SYMPTOMS

The stages, their titles, and most of these symptoms come from "Diagnosis and Treatment of Pneumonitis with a New Coronavirus Infection."[28] Most of the rest of the descriptions come from the Louisiana ER doctor. Since originally writing this section it has become increasingly difficult to keep to a stage-by-stage outline, since there are so many variable presentations. However, this still seems helpful for visualizing the process.

"Clinical Observation Stage"

The original Chinese account of coronavirus symptoms started with symptoms rather typical of the flu: fatigue with gastrointestinal discomfort, fatigue with fever. This is an observational stage, as the condition may be an ordinary flu.[29]

Stage 1: "Early Stage"

The Louisiana ER doctor writes: "2–11 days after exposure (day 5 on average) flu-like symptoms start." Symptoms: cold, dampness and functional depression; fever or no fever; dry cough, itchy throat, chest tightness; nausea without vomiting; fatigue; back pain (myalgia); abdominal discomfort with diarrhea in some cases; loss of sense of smell and taste, loss of appetite. The tongue is pale, pink, or red; the fur is white, thick, and sticky.[30]

Stage 2: "Plague Closes the Lungs"

Symptoms: persistent body heat or cold (chills) and fever, nasal congestion, sore, dry, itchy throat, dry cough, cough with little sputum, or yellow or bloody sputum, bloating and constipation, chest tightness, shortness of breath, coughing, relief, tongue body is red with a greasy, yellow coating, and the pulse is slippery.[31] Many people seem to jump from 0 to a 100 symptom-wise. Others do not.

Stage 3: "Severe Period"

The Louisiana ER doctor wrote: "Day 10—81% mild symptoms, 14% severe symptoms requiring hospitalization, 5% critical." Also: "Patient presentation is varied. Patients are coming in hypoxic (even 75%) without dyspnea. I have seen COVID patients present with encephalopathy, renal failure from dehydration, DKA. I have seen the bilateral interstitial pneumonia on the xray of the asymptomatic shoulder dislocation or on the CTs of the (respiratory) asymptomatic poly-trauma patient. Essentially if they are in my ER, they have it. Seen three positive flu swabs in 2 weeks and all three had COVID-19 as well. Somehow this . . . has told all other disease processes to get out of town."

Respiratory Presentation

This description reflects earlier accounts of the pandemic. Titles and symptoms come from the Chinese source: dyspnea, shortness of breath or asthmatic ventilation, unconsciousness, irritability, cold sweaty limbs, dark purple tongue, thick greasy or dry fur, large pulses without roots. The dark purple tongue (see two case histories in the liver section) indicates severe blood coagulation and fits with the following description.

Circulatory Presentation

An article in the *Washington Post*, summarizing scientific sources, was reprinted by the *Minneapolis Star Tribune*.[32] This rounded up the following symptoms as now characteristic: strokes from blood clots; neurological issues; pinkeye; loss of smell and taste; unexpected blood clotting; damage to lining of blood vessels; vomiting and diarrhea; clogged and inflamed alveoli (air sacs), hampering breathing; pulmonary embolism from blood clots, and microbes; weakened heart muscle; arrhythmias and heart attacks; damage to structures that filter waste from the blood; purple rash on toes or fingers from the attack on blood vessels; widespread immune-system impact, including an overactive immune response that attacks healthy tissue (the often fatal "cytokine storm").

The article asks whether this new symptomology represented an evolution of the disease or our understanding? This question is answerable. An autopsy on three patients who died in the 2003 SARS epidemic showed the same kind of damage.[33] The dark purple tongue noted in the respiratory description indicates blood stasis.

Stage 4: "Recovery Period"

You made it, you're alive, but you are exhausted and depleted. Symptoms: shortness of breath (now from exhaustion and damage, not closure), fatigue, anorexia, nausea, fullness, thin stools, pale tongue and greasy fur, unpleasant bowel evacuation. The pale tongue indicates depletion of blood or *qi* (nerve energy to push the blood to the surface).[34]

TEMPERATURE AND MOISTURE

Traditional herbalism is largely based on the doctrine of humoralism or "energetics" whereby one attempts to determine whether the person is hot or cold, damp or dry, tense or relaxed. Then the remedy or formula is administered "by contrary" (hot to cold), so that, for example, Ginger dried or fresh is warming to a "cold stomach," and Peach is cooling. In terms of the energetics of COVID: People can tell from their desires for warmth or cooling which of these two most important energetics they need.

Warming or Cooling?

COVID seems to produce little temperature at first; perhaps there will be a slight chill. In others there is a severe chill. Many people therefore need warming medicines. As the condition progresses, but sometimes perhaps from the start, there may be a need for cooling medicines.

The case history from Italy (see p. 117) demonstrates the importance of warming medicines and the detriment from cold. Here is one of the few case histories that show the symptom "better from cooling."

> **Case History, Elizabeth:** *Elizabeth had "chest heaviness in the bottom of the lungs." I am "Experimenting with Rosa damascena essential oil in jojoba on the chest for the lungs/pneumonia symptoms, as I think Lomatium is too hot for me and I do not have Nigella. Decided to approach COVID-19 from its angry center and see if this could be energetically helpful, as I am looking for another herb in the cabinet to help." Cinquefoil was beneficial. During her recuperation she took warming herbs, especially Angelica.*[35]

Cooling remedies include fruity plants such as Elderberry, Rose, Hawthorn, Peach, Lemon, and Lime. The latter two are also alkalinizing.

Elderberry *(Sambucus nigra, S. canadensis).* This the most famous herbal antiviral and is widely touted as a preventative and treatment for colds and flus. There is some scientific evidence for this, but application for prevention of COVID is unproven. Early in the epidemic it came under fire for possibly exaggerating the "cytokine storm" that is a factor in severe cases of coronavirus, according to experts. This theory is fatuous and is solidly rebutted by Stephen Harrod Buhner in *Herbal Antivirals: Natural Remedies for Emerging & Resistant Viral Infections* (2013). He recommends extraction from the leaves for more potency; most herbalists use the flowers (which are diaphoretic—open the skin) or berries. I feel Elderberry should seldom be used in cold cases since the flower is quite cooling and the berry somewhat. There are mixed reviews of the effectiveness of Elderberry or Elder Flower at this time.

Chinese Skullcap *(Scutellaria baicalensis).* Used in a formula with Forsythia and Honeysuckle, this medicinal plant has been highly recommended for COVID-19 in China. Honeysuckle *(Lonicera spp.)* is a cousin of Elderberry. American cousins Skullcap *(Scutellaria laterifolia)* or Lemon Balm *(Melissa officinalis)* may be fair substitutes. Several people were taught about Skullcap in dream or vision. Here is an amusing example. Skullcap is cooling.

> **Case History, Lizzie:** *In a plant journey during the winter, prior to the coronavirus epidemic, "a Chinese man came and placed a skullcap on my head and said I would be needing that. I wasn't sure why I would need a new hat, so I googled 'China skullcap,' discovered it was an actual plant with all its rich qualities, ordered a tincture, and now realize it was the main remedy I personally needed for COVID-19. It has met me so well, I truly think it has been integral in fighting off this virus for me when it went deeper and my weakened immune system struggled."*[36]

Rose Petals, Hips. Rose is cooling; it is recommended when the heat is penetrating past the superficial level (indicated by carmine or pink-red mucosa and complexion) to a deeper level, indicated by darker red color (when the complexion or tongue shows a mixture of carmine and dark red). Dandelion Root is also indicated for dark red mucosa and tongue.

Here is a case where the person overused warming remedies.

Case History, Mike: *A correspondent on Facebook writes, "I finally tested positive about 10 days in since symptoms slowly came on. It was so suppressed and dry that it felt like a tickle almost until it moved deeper into my lungs, never once becoming wet or depressed except in my throat.*

"I made the major mistake of overheating my center and drying myself out, which aggravated and atrophied my lungs and chest to an ongoing painful experience.

"I've since moved to a combo of Lemon Balm, Rose, and Borage [mucilaginous, cooling], with Mallow and Mullein. Pleurisy Root in very small-drop doses when I feel any airway wheezing or dry constriction. Mostly because all of these are in my garden and my apothecary wasn't very well stocked for this.

"I've kept up with a nitric oxide supplement and heavy A and D vitamins, occasionally adding Reishi back into the mix in moderate doses."

A white, adhesive coating and (sometimes) a pale tongue indicate a cold condition. Employ strategies to thin and disperse the fluids, warm the interior, and increase circulation (Lomatium, Angelica, Thyme, Fenugreek, Nigella, Bayberry Bark, Helichrysum, Garlic, Onions, Cayenne, Turmeric). Keep the skin open (Yarrow, Hyssop, Pleurisy Root, Elder Flower), and bowels open (Fenugreek, Yellow Dock Root). Yarrow is normalizing between warming and cooling. Conifer resins are stimulating and expectorant, such as Pine (bark or needles), Black Spruce (traditional Ojibwa cold remedy), White Spruce (tea opens the upper chest).

Tulsi *(Ocimum sanctum).* The government of India recommends frequent sipping of water boiled with tulsi as a general remedy for

COVID.[37] This herb is moderately warming and considered detoxifying.

Angelica *(Angelica archangelica),* **Lomatium** *(Lomatium dissectum),* **Osha Root** *(Ligusticum porteri).* These "Bear Medicines" (oily, warm, spicy, stimulating, drying) are some of the most important remedies, in my opinion and experience. They increase circulation, perhaps reducing blood pressure and blood coagulation. In the recuperation phase they have proved helpful to some—"Bear Medicines" give stamina. It is available from the liquor store in the liqueur Benedictine.

Sweet or Life Everlasting *(Helichrysum spp., Gnapalium spp.).* Members of the everlasting clan have three traits suited to COVID: they are traditional cold remedies (the coronavirus clan is a major source for this condition), they are used for both bruising and hemorrhaging, and reputedly lessen scar tissue. I have been recommending them for COVID-19, and now I find that there may be a good pharmacological basis for this. *Surviving Coronavirus,* by Su Fairchild, M.D. (2020), mentions a study in which helichrysetin, a constituent of *Helichrysum odoratissimum,* has been found to be active against various coronaviruses. This study dates to before the current novel-coronavirus.[38] I have three reports from people using Rabbit Tobacco or Helichrysum in the recuperation phase—all reported better respiration.

Moistening or Drying?

The Chinese doctor Liu Lihong (introduced above) comments, "Almost everyone agrees that dampness is at the core of this disease. All of the cases we have encountered so far display a thick, white, sticky tongue coating." But then he adds something interesting that may refer to the environment. "Since our arrival in Wuhan, every one of us has observed an increase in sticky coating on our own tongues, as well as the onset of incomplete bowel movements." Confirmation from the pulse: "Virtually everyone exhibits a slippery pulse" in the lung position, confirming that "turbid damp obstructing the Lung is the main characteristic of this epidemic." This may be the presentation in cool, damp climates or it may be more universal. The virus seems to be highly adaptable. Many people feel dry rather than damp, but that can mean that fluids are stuck inside and not coming out. Others definitely feel hot.

Mucus is a form of dampness. When it dries out we use mucilages or moistening substances to get the mucous membranes hydrated and healthy. Many people seem to need moistening remedies, others need the drying, or different remedies are needed in different stages. The "Bear Medicines" I have been recommending—Lomatium, Osha, and Angelica—can be drying.

Mucilage is a slimy, mucus-like constituent found in many plants. We frequently use Marshmallow Root and Slippery Elm in herbal medicine. Onion syrup, mentioned elsewhere, is warming and slimy. Mucilaginous foods include oats, okra, and flax seed.

Licorice. *Glycorrhiza spp.* is an immune-modulating mucilage that is being used in a lot of the Chinese formulae and by Western practitioners. I have stayed away from it because it can cause high blood pressure, which would not be good here.

Fenugreek. My favorite mucilage for COVID is *Trigonella foenum-graecum.* It is warming, soothing, lubricating, oily, moist, and expectorant; it is frequently used in Middle Eastern, Ayurvedic, Chinese, and Western herbalism. Fenugreek and Thyme is a favorite combination for colds and flus.

Solomon's Seal *(Polygonatum spp.).* Not to be confused with the Smartweed clan *(Polygonum),* this medicine plant is usually used to lubricate tendons and ligaments but can be used as a mucilage.

Case History, Lise: *Herbalist Lise Wolf sent me a case history from one of her students.[39] "A few years ago I gave my friend Aaron a spray bottle of Solomon's Seal for repetitive stress injury (he's a bartender and had severe pain in his elbow and forearm for awhile). The Solomon's Seal worked well for him (in combination with Agrimony). Then the other day he told me that when he recently contracted coronavirus (he didn't get tested but all the symptoms checked out) he started using the Solomon's Seal as a throat spray,* *once in the morning and once at night. He said he 'couldn't breathe well because of the gunk in my lungs' but that the Solomon's Seal helped him breathe more easily."*

Formula for sticky phlegm, thickened fluids: Pleurisy Root, Yerba Mansa, Red Root, Bayberry Bark. Warming mucilages to coat the membranes: Fenugreek, Onion. Phyllis Light, whom I consider a master in the field, has been "using a combination of Bayberry, Yarrow, and Cayenne."[40]

SYMPTOMS, SYSTEMS, AND HERBS

Traditional herbal medicine attempts to strengthen the body to resist the contagion or disease, or to recover from the insult or injury, on its own. This, we believe, leads to long-term health. We do not oppose well-thought-out medical intervention.

When we don't fully understand the underlying pathology we study the symptomology and attempt to address these, as evidence of the "inner cries" of the body for help in certain regions, functions, or situations.

Onset

Most people are chilly—warm yourself up as quickly as possible. Use warm water, if nothing else is available. Warming kitchen herbs such as Rosemary, Thyme, Turmeric, Ginger, and Cayenne may be beneficial.

Case History, Lizzie (continued): *"It was sudden, like flu can be, where within an hour or two you're suddenly struck with ice-cold shaking chills, rigours, everything dysregulated: that state where you find yourself making sickly moaning noises to yourself and wondering who is making that pitiful noise; that felt sense that it is fast consuming you, that something has gone deep deep, and that you can't control what is happening with your body . . . it hit my heart,* *lungs, upper chest like an invisible yet tangible being, and I felt like I was breathing in toxic fumes, even though at that stage my breathing was fine . . . like something noxious to me was consuming. My heart was tachycardic and intense and dysregulated."*

Anxiety and Fear

A friend of mine went into a coffee shop he noticed was open during the lockdown. He could get coffee but not sit down. The owner said, "You've heard of flight-or-fight?" Yeah, answered my friend. "Well, all the flight people are at home; all the fight people are the ones that come in." See the homeopathic and flower essences remedies mentioned above for anxiety and fear. Several case histories also refer to the fear.

Case History, Lizzie (continued): *"There was a sense of embodied fear. I knew in the moment it was serious and that it was something my body didn't understand but was very alarmed about. At that point I had not even considered at all that it was COVID-19, just that something was seriously amiss. The fear wasn't an anticipatory fear about being ill, it was more that the illness feels like it holds or triggers an energy of fear, in the same way that Lyme seems to embody/trigger a dark destructive energy."*

Psycho-Spiritual Changes

One characteristic symptom of COVID is the number of people who are having dreams, hunches, and visions, often about what to do. Several of us believe this is characteristic of a positive response to the virus, and that people should follow these subjective experiences. Herbalist and therapist Mary Pat Palmer comments, "I can tell you as a therapist that when people start dreaming about their problems this is an excellent indication of health and an important way to process life issues." It is very important, therapeutically, to acknowledge this element of COVID. This is demonstrated by a comment on my personal Facebook page (May 24, 2020): "As a psychotherapist in Humboldt County, working with Veterans, I have observed an increase in reporting of significant dreams, who described new 'atrial fibrillation' and other possible COVID-19 symptoms, but were not treated by medical providers." This may lead to "possible self-awareness for treatment" of the virus.

Many people have had meaningful dreams relating to COVID, the meaning of their symptoms, herbs to take, ancestors, family, spiritual issues, or even the relationship between humanity, the Earth, and COVID.[41] Lizzie, for example, dreamed that she was being attacked by a shark with the name "Covid the 19th" written on the side: "It seems the gods were really trying to make me wake up and see what was happening; this was not a time for subtle metaphors." I personally had a dream every single time anything COVID-related occurred in my system—over twenty instances. This included the virus showing me that it attacked the dreaming centers in the brain. This connection led herbalist Phyllis Light to the use of pineal-strengthening herbs and foods, since this gland is related to sleep and dream. Unfortunately, not much is known about herbs for this gland. Phyllis' foremost remedy, based on the doctrine of signatures, is Pine; the pineal was named due to its visual similarity to a pinecone.

The following case, which gained some notoriety,[42] shows deep psycho-spiritual changes, but this may be due to the near-death experience rather than the direct influence of the virus.

Case History, Titou Phommachanh: *Age 44. High blood pressure was the only pre-existing condition. This is a well-documented case because his wife went to the media to get the test and experimental drug (remdesiver) that may or may not have saved his life. He had the characteristic double pneumonia. He was put on a ventilator, but that wasn't enough so he was put in an induced coma for two weeks, and given a lung bypass (oxygenating the blood in a machine while his lungs recover). They call his room the "good luck room" since another young man survived with the lung bypass in that room.*

Katie Walsh was the caregiver after he was discharged as not contagious. "We did some Old World steams. Fresh Pine needles and cones. Tried Lobelia. I feel like I should have taken Skullcap with me, but I didn't." Lobelia helped him sweat.

"He was totally changed by the disease. He was never an emotional person. His wife, my cousin, did most of the talking for him. Now he is 'emotionally there,' comment his friends. He had a life-changing experience. He saw his life flash before his mind from beginning to end; he saw his girls in the future without him. Now he is incredibly attentive. He feels he survived for a purpose, although he also has survivor's guilt."

Titou had a vision during the induced coma that was the one thing he remembered from that time: "He was a fish out of water and he had the choice to enter a flowing stream where he would have died, but he chose to stay alive on earth and survive. He chose to be with his kids." Unfortunately, he is still deeply traumatized from waking from a coma at night, alone, in a hospital bed in restraints.

"His tastes for food totally changed. He couldn't tolerate processed food, basically. He only eats fruit and Laotian stew."

The following case has some similarities to this one.

Encephalopathy

I am going to leave out the discussion, prevention, and treatment of stroke (from the blood clotting) as too serious for this article. Other brain-related presentations occur. "It is reported that CoV can be found in the brain or cerebrospinal fluid."[43]

Case History, Christine (continued): *"So I'm still dealing with what my ER doctor friend believes to be the neurological subset version of COVID. Good times! Not. I've been getting out of bed for an hour a few times a day yesterday and today so that is an improvement! I'm on a second wave of it as I thought I was just getting over the* *hump the first time when I was hit again with a round wave. So it is improving. Both CNS and PNS involvement—really not nice headaches, dizziness, nausea, hard to think and focus, tingling and numbness, hyper sensorial sensitivity, body is racing, wired but tired, shaky, weak, rolling sensations moving through my body and brain, vibrating and spinning chakras, keep losing vasovagal tone, skin is sore, thermo-dysregulation, neuroendocrine dysfunction so things likely hypoglycemia, excessive hunger but still significant weight loss. (No excessive thirst or urination.) Mild GI upset. I used to think the joke that 'we are all just one good flu away from our ideal weight' was funny. There is a feeling that the whole world is closing in on and around me.*

"Night time offers no reprieve as I'm bombarded by disincarnated beings that have died but they did not know they died as they were heavily sedated to go on ventilators. So when they wake up they think they have survived. I'm having to tell them their body did not make it. It is so upsetting and disturbing to say the least. So in short, I feel like I have been in an ayahuasca ceremony for two weeks straight now and around the clock.

"I was completely unprepared for this subset of COVID! I felt pretty prepared and was having success working with the respiratory version! Relaxing nervines were not helpful alone. When I moved to adding adaptogens it calmed things down a bit, so less wired now. Phew! Ganoderma, Withania, Hypericum, Scutellaria, are some other herbs in my formula. I can't remember the rest right now. Taking B Complex and Omega 3."

Neurological Effects

In addition to the effects on the brain there can be effects on the rest of the nervous system. We see the effects on the peripheral (sensory) with the changes in smell and taste; on the autonomic with regard to the vagus and diaphragm, in charge of breathing, and in many other regions (see Sara Annon's case history on page 144).

Case History, Titou Phommachanh (continued): *Katie Walsh described the symptoms she observed and amended after Titou left the hospital: "The whole arm was tingly. The last three fingers were relentlessly painful, tingling, annoying. I gave him massages with Yarrow, a spritzer of Yarrow, and soaked his hand in Yarrow and Lobelia infusion, but the Lobelia internally. That seemed to help, along with Turmeric tablets his wife gave."*

Loss of Sense of Smell and Taste

It is now well known that a complete loss of smell and taste may be an early warming sign of coronavirus, which in some cases strikes directly at the olfactory nerve at the roof of the nose, just between the eyes. One of my friends had this symptom *only,* lasting for over a month, until she consulted an experienced herbalist.[44]

Red Eyes, Burning Tears

These symptoms are recorded by many. There is some question whether this is due to irritation of the eyes or an emotional component of the disease. One friend had this symptom for over six weeks.

Throat

An itchy, irritated sore throat is highly characteristic and can carry on throughout the epidemic. I have heard it said that "the virus lives in the throat"; this fits the experience of many.

There are two basic types of sore throat: (1) swollen glands, usually palpable and often painful on swallowing, and (2) irritation of the vagus resulting in irritable membranes without the above symptoms. Both can occur in COVID and other acute diseases. A standard remedy for the former is Cleavers *(Galium aparine)* and for the latter:

Nigella sativa **(Black Seed, Black Cumin)** is a well-rounded, exhaustively studied immune tonic with an ancient pedigree.[45] Research shows that it covers just about all the typical regions affected by COVID: lungs, heart, digestive tract, liver, kidneys, nervous system. (It is contraindicated in pregnancy.) This agent (with Holly and Lomatium, and Fenugreek) helped me for weeks. Every time I had a sore throat I took the raw seeds and it disappeared within ten minutes. It settles irritation of the vagus or autonomic nervous system, which COVID may be attacking elsewhere in the body.

Lungs

The infection goes down from the throat to the trachea and bronchia. There is often a dry, itchy sensation and cough, with weight on the chest. Breathlessness can occur in the first minutes and disappear or remain or come and go. As the symptoms get worse the mucus and dampness build up. A distinctive feature is the absence of expectoration of the phlegm. Liu Lihong[46] says that this causes "turbid phlegm to congeal into a rubbery and glue-like material that severely interferes with proper airway function and has no way out." He concludes, "This is the most important reason for the lingering 'stalemate' quality of the disease, as well as the tendency to take a sudden turn for the worse."

Case History, Amy: *"I think I had this thing coming off a Caribbean cruise March 15th. It took me out for 3½ weeks! Prickles in throat, dry cough, and breathlessness. No fever. I used lung tea, which helped significantly. Ingredients: Mullein, Marshmallow Root, Osha Root, Licorice Root, and Yerba Santa. Also [kinesiology testing indicated I take] Pleurisy Root, Red Root, Elecampane and Hyssop as well as (oddly enough) Prickly Ash tincture every few days and Hawthorn almost every day.*

"Ultimately I used my hubby's inhaler once at the end to push open the bronchia as an acupuncturist friend advised—that really helped push me into being better because the hardest part was feeling like I could complete breaths; otherwise I was virtually fine. It would be like that for over a week. I thought I was better and then I wouldn't be able to complete breaths fully.

"Oddly my hubby was only sick 4 days and he has asthma bad.

He took steroids when we got off the ship and he drank 3 gallons a day of the tea [above]. It was so weird because he had all the symptoms I did.

"I got sick after he got well. I haven't been sick in over 20 years with flu. Hypothyroid, low adrenals, and anemia—yes—but no colds or flus."

Mullein (*Verbascum thapsus, V. spp.*). Coronavirus erodes the cilia (hairs) in the lungs: Three herbs I know of protect those tiny, brushy hairs—Mullein, Horsetail, and Comfrey. Many strains of Comfrey contain pyrrolizidine alkaloids and should not be used in COVID, if possible, due to the liver involvement.

Case History, anonymous: *"I have all the COVID symptoms and had recent regional travel to big events. We've been tested by public health but tests came back negative (apparently this was quite common in China too). However, what has helped me the most is Mullein. I haven't been able to get any Elecampane, but Mullein is pretty common. I drank the simple tea (steeped for at least 15 minutes) every 2–4 hrs while awake and that has helped with the chest tightness. Oddly enough it seems to work best on its own without cayenne and with a pinch of sugar; I'm not sure why the sugar helps I can't even taste it. Maybe it's available where you are. It also helps with the GI manifestations, or it's helped me anyways."*[47]

Sugar is a mild relaxant to the throat and lungs—excellent for hiccoughs. Mullein works best in hot infusion because water extracts the salty mucilage (the part we want), which can be seen floating on the surface.

Case History, Chris M.: *An herbalist friend went to the hospital at the peak of his infection to get a chest x-ray. He had viral double pneumonia and hypoxia down to 91%. The physicians diagnosed*

COVID on the symptoms, as tests were not yet available. That night he woke with an intense bolt of fear running through him. He immediately felt it was not his own emotion, rejected it, and it left him. From that night on he started to get better. I called him about something else shortly after and recommended Mullein since his cilia were inflamed. He had some on hand and got relief during the pneumonia from Mullein tea hourly, as well as tincture. "After I could walk from one room to the other I starting taking Osha Root and about a day later it provoked the suppressed cough reflex."

Prickly Ash Bark (*Xanthoxylum americanum*). This extremely stimulating medicinal plant is an important remedy to rally the resistance in serious bronchitis.[48] It increases circulation to the capillary bed. It also is stimulating to the nervous system but not exactly warming—for those who need a stimulant but not too much heat. Nicole Duxbury used it in several cases.[49]

Yerba Mansa. Early, before COVID was an epidemic in the US, herbalist Michael Cottingham and I talked about the importance of this remedy (*Amenopsis californica*). It is for boggy, waterlogged tissues, especially in the upper and lower respiratory tract. We thought of combining it with Pleurisy Root (*Asclepias tuberosa*). He found a good combination was with Rosemary (*Rosmarinus officinalis*).

Onion Syrup. Chop an Onion and place the pieces in maple syrup or honey. This will draw out the mucilage and warming volatile oils to create a respiratory syrup that moistens and loosens phlegm and stimulates a healthy cough. Similar to Yerba Santa in properties, but more readily available.[50]

Pine Needles, Pine Bark (*Pinus strobus, P. spp.*). This warming aromatic herb has long been used in herbal medicine to bring up difficult-to-raise phlegm and is widely available. Positive reports have come in.[51]

Note: A Cough that is Not COVID. I had a hard time telling the difference between the cough of COVID and the dry, irritable cough that is typical in dry winter air or from forced-air furnaces and wood stoves, so I think this is important to point out. Marshmallow Root at night, just before bed (many other herbalists do this too), palliates. American or California Spikenard (*Aralia racemosa, A. Californica*) was more specific for me. It would take it away altogether. If one can't get the herb get the homeopathic (Aralia 6x, 6c).

Hypoxia

This is a medical condition, not a symptom. Most people are unaware that they are suffering from hypoxia (low oxygen levels in the blood). This is one of the most important indications of a serious COVID condition, since it leads to both respiratory and circulatory problems. Therefore, *one of the best instruments to have on hand is a pulse oximeter,* which quickly, inexpensively, and easily measures this in the home.

Herbalists including Lisa Ganora and Leslie Alexander early on were using Rhodiola, an astringent "adaptogen" well-known for altitude sickness (naturally occurring hypoxia). This herb is used in the Chinese formulas for COVID. Garlic may be a simple home remedy for this condition.

Heart

My early drafts for this article described "the metaphorical heart" because there was no information on damage to the physical heart. The first reports of arrhythmias and ischemias (heart attacks) came to me from personal correspondence, not popular or professional news. These terrible pathological occurrences were then confirmed in a *Scientific American* article.[52] Initial evidence indicates that the virus can directly attack the heart, which also contains ACE2 receptors, and that this happens in as many as one in five cases. Later the problem with blood coagulation was discovered.

My first symptom (March 8) was rapid heartbeat (140–150 per minute), which would surely damage the heart had it not been stopped in five minutes by application of Lomatium tincture in repeated doses (probably about five or eight "squirts" of the tincture). I also experienced an attack on my "metaphorical heart:" COVID seemed to hang over me like a dark ectoplasm beaming hatred at me. When I asked it "why do you hate me so much?" it replied clear as a human voice: "I'm everything you hate." Thereafter I took Holly (the flower essence for feeling hate or being hated) as well as Lomatium. They always caused the circulation in my chest to expand, as if the heart, upper lungs, and thymus (immune gland) were being protected by release of blood pressure and a myriad of immune cells.

"This virus goes straight to the heart," writes Minneapolis herbalist Nicole Duxbury. "I do believe it asks us to process unprocessed emotions (collective or personal). Part of my healing involved waves of deep grief (came on co-with symptoms each time)."[53]

Case History, Lizzie (continued): *"Rapidly I went through incredible sickness with chest compressed by great weight, like a vice was tightening around chest, extreme tachycardia, simply from moving an arm or trying to reach for water. Angina, heart randomly slowing, halting, and rebounding. Extreme breathlessness due to heart— not lungs. Huge painful swelling of lymph glands in and around left armpit when body was fighting the infection with all its resilience and might around heart area, with all the associated fevers and chills and poorliness. Much erratic arrythmia, and slightest slightest movement causing all the above to worsen. It reminded me of Lyme carditis only this was far worse, far more systemic. It felt, without wishing to sound dramatic, 'threatening' . . . and messages in my shamanic journeys to 'take this very seriously and not underestimate this, this is viral myocarditis,' made me stop . . . and so I lay there and breathed slow and deep and kept repeating 'I can expand to hold all of this' then oscillated into good old-fashioned mortal fallible fear and late-night texts to friends asking them to confirm I would live and if I didn't that I loved them lots.*

"And so I journeyed deeper and deeper each hour to find out

how to meet this, what my body needed. In early days homeopathic Digitalis helped shift a layer, then I remembered Cactus grandiflorus tincture (which had really helped after Lyme weakened valves) in single drops, taken under tongue now and then and smoothed regularly up my heart meridian and armpit glands. Cactus eased the vise around my chest, and angina type state. Aurum [homeopathic gold] briefly came alongside and met and cleared at an emotional level: big old dark night of the soul heart feeling states. But after several days or a week homeopathic Spigelia did the biggest physical shift, so much so that I cried in amazement at the little sugar pills' power. Within a few doses everything began to shift to the point where after a few days I no longer felt like there is any infection affecting heart, all painful gland swelling completely went. Now my heart is now simply tired and weak, as am I.

"All the way through I was having hawthorn flower/leaf/berry/thorn tincture, which I have been having daily since it finished brewing last autumn. I added in some Motherwort when heart first went poorly fast, it was and still is a reassuring soothing nourishing ally but didn't feel like alone it would have met this acute illness state."

Hawthorn. The first remedy that comes to mind for the heart for most herbalists would be Hawthorn (*Crataegus* spp.), a first cousin of the apple and entirely safe. It appears to increase circulation to both the periphery (taking pressure off the heart) and the heart itself (to feed, nourish, and cleanse). It also has a regulatory effect on cholesterol, though that would not be needed in acute conditions. This effect can be increased by the addition of Solomon's Seal (*Polygonatum* spp.), which loosens tendons and ligaments in the chest. As little as seven parts Hawthorn to one part Solomon's Seal will work—which is a good thing, since the latter is in short supply.

Holly. This is widely available as the Bach Flower Essence Holly (*Ilex opaca*), which is used for hatred and fear. I have also made tincture or tea from the leaves—the berries are a ferocious purgative that should not be used. The dose need only be a few drops, as needed, or a few times a day.

I first began to use this remedy for the extreme fatigue that accompanies Bartonella, one of the Lyme co-infections, and I found it successful in three cases, including my own. I took Holly because of the way Bartonella (diagnosed by a professional from the symptoms) attacked my brain and heart within days of the bite. This is similar to COVID, and I have been using this remedy for myself and recommending it for others when the "heart felt attacked," i.e., by pressure on the upper chest. One of the few other herbalists who uses Holly, to my knowledge, is Amanda Dilday. It turned out she too was applying it for COVID exactly as I was.[54]

When a plant looks like an animal or is used by an animal, it is classified as an "animal medicine" in Native American herbalism.[55] Holly qualifies in both capacities as a "Bat Medicine" because of the way the thorns on the leaves look like the claws on a bat's wing; and the bats will make their homes in the dark interior of the little tree. Bats are the ultimate source of COVID. Because they have a highly efficient immune system, viruses have to mutate quickly in order to establish themselves. When such a virus moves to a human being it retains this reproductive rapidity and, perhaps, mutability.

Amanda sees a resemblance between the way bats sense in the darkness by sonar (signals emanating out and coming back) and the way the heart senses in the darkness of emotional uncertainty. Bats are creepy, yes, but they are loving parents who carefully raise, feed, and train their young.[56]

Rosemary (*Rosmarinus officinalis*). This warming, drying, stimulating herb has an effect on the circulation and nervous system generally, so it indirectly supports the cardiovascular and respiratory systems.

From a therapeutic standpoint, the remedies to prevent hemorrhaging and blood coagulation fall into several categories. Blood stagnation is eminently treatable by the same kinds of warming stimulants and resinous warming plants for which "damp stagnation" can be approached (Lomatium, Angelica, Yarrow, Cinnamon, etc.).

Gastrointestinal Presentation

From a medical writer in March 2020: "Novel coronavirus symptoms seem to be mostly focused on fever and cough, but gastrointestinal symptoms should be a new focus for clinicians, according to two new papers published online in *Gastroenterology*."[57, 58] In these cases the ACE2 receptor cells in the intestines showed signs of COVID entry. Characteristic symptoms include: diarrhea, nausea, vomiting, abdominal discomfort; loose or constipated, frequency and unpleasant smell; passing gas; changes in bowel habits.

If the symptoms tend toward cold and damp (gurgling, diarrhea) try warming remedies (dried Ginger, Angelica, Smartweed, etc.). If there is spasm (nausea, vomiting, constipation), warming agents may help but relaxants like Nigella, Peppermint, and Magnesium may assist.

Liver Presentation

Evidence shows that COVID patients are affected in the liver. Moderate cases show some elevated enzymes, but fatal cases often show high levels. One woman (with pre-existing conditions) presented with acute hepatitis as the main symptom.[59]

In Western herbalism the word *liver* is used in a metaphorical sense to represent the metabolism in general. In Chinese herbalism *liver* refers to harmonious movement of energy in the system (i.e., tension). Since energy ("qi") moves blood, the severe symptoms of COVID with the purple tongue and blood stagnation can be associated with the liver. A chief symptom of liver East or West is anger ("binding of the qi"). Intense chills and fever are also associated with the liver and gallbladder. Practitioners may see a combination of these physical and metaphorical symptoms.

Case History posted by acupuncturist Julia Brodzinski, L.Ac.:[60] *"I definitely experienced firsthand how useful Bupleurum is when the cold damp stagnation starts to generate some heat, which I saw in the progression of a very pale, puffy tongue to the development of slightly* *dusky, slightly purple sides. Also the cycling back and forth between feeling well and then another relapse, between symptoms that worsen and then appear at different times in the day, fevers that come and go—since these are key indications for Bupleurum it really seemed like it was a good match. I hesitated to use it when there were only cold and damp symptoms because I didn't want to aggravate either the cold or the damp with cold herbs. But once the shift to a deeper level with even just a little heat occurred, it worked amazingly well.*

"There were a lot of other herbs in the formula I used, 14 actually, each playing an important role in moving through the stagnant damp, venting the heat, draining the damp, healing inflammation in the lungs, harmonizing the digestion, and also fighting the virus directly. But one challenge I found with using Bupleurum so aggressively is that it can be very depleting, and I had left out the traditional ginseng and jujube dates from the formula that counteract this effect, because of the risk of creating more stagnation and because I wanted to make sure the viral infection was gone before tonifying."

I have seen a solidly purple tongue only once ("stroke" was the diagnosis, though he got so much better under Sassafras tincture that I concluded he just had "thick blood"—his pulse felt like oatmeal). When I visited the following case on the first day she had purple sides to her tongue (relieved only temporarily with Lomatium and Yarrow). She had far to go.

Case History, Sara Annon: *My friend had a brain injury and scar tissue throughout her body and liver from, among other things, a lightning strike. She writes articulately.[61] I left out the cranial symptoms and focused her account on the liver and GI symptoms.*

"Horsetail tincture has been able to interrupt the cycle of ever-increasing inflammation for me. Just a drop or two several times a day soothes and strengthens my tissues, reducing inflammation and increasing circulation. Then the old, putrid, toxic and coarse matter

causing the inflammation could be eliminated, I hoped. To my frustration, my body simply did not seem to have the resources to actually bring things to a head and expel the unwanted material.

"I suspect the irritability of an inflamed vagus nerve was part of the paroxysms of vomiting, especially since there was no nausea involved. I also had not considered the details of how the vagus nerve affects liver function. I know that under stress, my entire digestive tract shuts down, and getting circulation and movement returned is a challenge. But until now, I had not realized that since bile ducts are made of smooth muscle with peristalsis just like the intestines, they would react with acute spasms when the rest of my guts do. Scarring and intra-hepatic blockages were already interfering with the circulation and elimination of blood, lymph, and bile in my liver.

"I celebrated Easter week with ever-larger swellings that could be described as hot boils, cold cysts and sterile abscesses popping up in most uncomfortable places. Swelling in my liver felt especially compromising, putting pressure on some of the major veins returning blood to the heart. By Good Friday, the tension in my body had built to the verge of incapacitating. But on Saturday, the pressure in my head abruptly broke once I stood up. I found myself spitting out mouthfuls of bloody serum and bone grit as I began to move around.

"This time the abrupt paroxysms in my smooth muscles were at least headed in the right direction. Instead of vomiting, swallowing set off sudden spasms and explosive diarrhea, which included the bile backed up in my liver bursting loose and being ejected along with any blockages.

"By noon, the recalcitrant boil on the inside of my upper thigh was about the size and shape of my thumb and it equally suddenly came to a head, painlessly releasing its plentiful quantity of pus. As the sun went down on Easter Sunday, I finally felt like my body would be capable of recuperating from this latest round of health challenges. I find the timing of my recent breakthrough serendipitous.

"Horsetail tincture has helped to reduce the inflammation in *my CNS. It is helping my system to repair my nerve sheaths and mucous membranes and strengthen my blood vessels so I have had less leakage from the AV [cranial] malformation. It has also soothed my spleen and kidneys as well as my liver enough that my edema is receding from dangerous extremes."* It is an old friend she had dreamed about in the past.

Herbal liver support includes St. John's Wort (also antiviral), Dandelion Root, Milk Thistle, Bupleurum, Agrimony, Cinquefoil, Blessed Thistle, and Camomile. Bupleurum is a very important liver remedy in Chinese herbalism. It has a reputation for bringing up deep emotional problems for which people are not always ready.

St. John's Wort (*Hypericum perforatum*). This well-known remedy is an antiviral that stimulates the CP450 pathway in the liver to help break down lipophilic toxins, so it may have an important part to play as an antiviral and a detoxifier. However, it can break down prescription drugs and should not be taken when a person is on many pharmaceuticals, including birth control.

Muscle and Bone Ache

Blood tests show that muscle tissue is being broken down quickly, causing the severe aches and pains typical of the flu that people are experiencing. This creates protein waste products that have to pass through the kidneys, forcing those organs to overwork. The urine may become dark and scanty or light and copious as the kidneys are stressed.

Boneset (*Eupatorium perfoliatum*). This is an old specific for flus and fevers where the bone ache is prominent or even severe, as if someone is breaking your bones. It is also for severe chills and intermittent fever and chill. Because it contains pyrrolizidine alkaloids, use drop doses (3–5 drops) or the homeopathic low potencies (6x, 6c, etc.). Lizzie reported that Boneset tincture in drop doses were her "main allies" for the "deep chills and fevers and pain like someone was breaking my ribs and spine bones." Chinese Skullcap stopped the "restlessness" and relaxed her system. She used Usnea (a mucilaginous lichen) when the symptoms were in the lungs.

Autonomic Nervous System

The autonomic (ANS) powers and regulates the involuntary functions of the body including digestion, circulation, respiration, blood pressure, and kidney and liver function, so it is clear that it is impacted by COVID just as are the central nervous system (CNS) and peripheral nervous system (senses). We treat the autonomic effectively in herbal medicine so this is important. The main nerve in the ANS is the vagus, which innervates the diaphragm—hence lung and stomach tension from excess and weakness from deficiency. I could not find discussion of the autonomic symptoms associated with COVID in scientific literature, but this was evident to practitioners—myself, Christine, and Sara. The passage of the ANS into the parasympathetic mode is required for immune health.

The upper reach of the vagus is in the back of throat and gives rise to some of the irritation felt there. I found this irritation ameliorated by Nigella. Sara commented on the vagal implications on the liver and gallbladder. Lizzie's description of fluctuating cardiac symptoms suggests vagal irregularity, and Christine commented on the vasovagal symptoms (blood volume changes) she experienced. A nurse Ph.D. described her presenting symptoms as "stuttering" in the respiratory nerves (CNS/ANS).

I believe Nigella is a good, safe agent for the autonomic (in addition to all its other wonder-effects), but not many people (except Middle Easterners) will have this on hand. Herbalists may have Lobelia, but this should not be used by non-professionals. These remedies will often relax the throat, diaphragm, and lungs. If the autonomic is weak, blood volume and heart rate may fluctuate, the person may gasp for breath from a weak diaphragm and compensate with abdominal muscles (which become sore). A remedy for both vagal tension and loss of tone is Agrimony (*Agrimonia* spp.) or its interchangeable cousin Cinquefoil (*Potentilla* spp.). In non-COVID presentations in years past I have seen

Agrimony work for "tortured to capture the breath," which is always accompanied by abdominal breathing.

Detoxification Headache and Bodyache

Although ignored in conventional medicine, everyone knows that a food, alcohol, or drug binge will be followed by a "hangover" with a dull, achy headache and achiness generally. This shows that the liver (and cells) are backed up with the job of catabolism or detoxification. This can be readily improved with herbs. Homeopathic Nux vomica 30x or 30c is excellent for these states.

Kidney Presentation

Death from kidney failure has not been reported, but harder work for the kidneys is a physiological necessity when tissue is being broken down and proteins have to be processed through them. In Chinese herbalism the kidneys are responsible for "grasping the qi in the lungs," or increasing the strength of inhalation. This seems to be a factor in COVID. Once a practitioner is trained to look for this, he or she will see it all the time.

Nettle. Judy Lieblein writes: "A lot of people have been craving Nettle lately, including people who generally don't drink it. I've been adding Linden so the mix isn't so drying. Linden is also beneficial for colds, flus, and helps with throats irritated from coughing."[62] Linden flowers are mucilaginous. This seems to be a remedy people are attracted to in the recuperation stage, when their kidneys are stressed. I have used Nettles in the past for sleep apnea; it increases iron and hemoglobin so the lungs can grasp more oxygen, and strengthening the kidneys—but is therefore drying to some.

Case History, Jessie Belden: *The Medicine Tree herb store, Minneapolis, writes, "The kidneys have been huge for me in this illness. Week one my kidneys were constantly aching—like they were being attacked! I started Nettle infusions with a pinch of*

marshmallow and licorice root and they were all better...still though,
the trouble with inhalation persisted. I have been on Cordyceps since
the beginning, but I have recently upped the dose and it seems to be
supporting the breath more.”[63]

Recuperation

Most of the advice here would be similar from one herbalist to another:
Patients should utilize easily digested, strengthening herbs. Also, take a
look at kidney and liver remedies if there is difficulty with detoxification. Astragalus and Codonopsis are in the Chinese formula for recovery. Gruel. Oatmeal. Slippery Elm Bark. Bioplasma (twelve cell salts).
Gentle circulatory stimulants are indicated. A number of people have
felt relief from Angelica. I personally felt noticeable improvement from
good quality, range-fed liver. Smartweed helped both Titou and myself.

Recuperation, Titou Phommachanh (continued): *Katie Walsh relates:*
“His mother couldn’t visit him directly but she instructed that he have
Smartweed, which was growing in the garden. I picked this—it was
the pink-flowered kind with an acrid taste—and gave him that in a
Laotian broth from his mother (chicken, rice, noodles, scallions, etc.).
That was all he wanted; he would eat it day and night. My cousin (his
wife) would get him everything he wanted; this was all he wanted.”[64]

Recuperation, Lizzie (continued): *“Little update, today my lungs*
feel like they are my own again—yay, no more breathlessness from
talking or just breathing . . . little by little shifting, changing.
*   “Last night in my journeys I was met by Bear and taken to the Arctic*
northern lands where he dug up roots for me: Burdock and Angelica—
new-to-me allies for this next phase of healing. He said they were for
replenishment, that this virus had deeply depleted [me], that my blood
needed both cleansing and rebuilding, that they would be strengthening
and the allies needed for this phase of healing and transformation.
I’ve never read about Burdock Root so I just did—how utterly

perfect for my dried-out atrophied now-toxic headachey-feeling self!

"Bear was very stern and clear that for 'those for whom this virus has gone deep, the period of convalescence is as vital a phase as any of the other phases and to be taken seriously. The virus depletes deeply, and transforms energy bodies and actual bodies, requiring deep deep sustained rest to replenish and adapt and realign into new form.'

"Bear also said that root medicine was needed at all stages but especially at convalescence: Oatstraw and Borage and other lovely things would not go deep enough, and again he lined up Burdock, Angelica, and added Astragalus for me, and nodded approvingly at my newfound craving for big bowls of Oats. And to keep homeopathic Cinchona close . . . and Cactus . . . still steadying my heart back to a balanced drumbeat, keeping her, the Queen of the Night [Cactus or Selenocereus grandiflors*], and Hawthorn by my side a while 'til I am strong."*

Smartweed (*Polygonum* spp.). Look for the species with pink flowers and a peppery taste—it is also called Water Pepper. One species is used in South Asian cooking. This is a fine stimulant, clears the mucosa of the respiratory and GI tracts. I personally benefited a great deal from this herb in my recuperation.

Burdock Root (*Arctium lappa*). This "Bear Medicine" provides oil that rebuilds the adrenal cortex (we think) and promotes steroid hormone production. It also helps with digestion and metabolism of fats and oils, according to herbal experience.

Angelica Root (*Angelica archangelica, Angelica* spp.). I've used this in cases where the lungs were full of water, the mind dull, the eyes bleary, after a bad bronchitis. It seems to improve stamina.

Oatstraw, Milky Oat Seed, and Oatmeal (*Avena sativa*). These are extremely convalescent in reputation and common experience. The first is more mineralizing; the latter two are somewhat mucilaginous (sticky and milky), also rich in minerals (if properly grown). People who are not diabetic may want to add maple syrup or some natural sweetening agent. Butter will help to replenish oils.

Contraindications

Some people cannot take immune tonics, blood-thinners, or St. John's Wort, so check for contraindications. Some even have an allergy to Garlic. Always test a remedy by taking a small dose first (this would even be a good idea with pharmaceutical drugs).

CONCLUSION

The article in *National Geographic* suggested that the intense dreams experienced by so many with COVID are due to social isolation and boredom. This is typical of conventional thinking, which ignores the subtle side of human existence. If we do not record our dreams, visions, hallucinations, and sensations from COVID, who will? I consider my article something of an historical document recording a few of these experiences. But it is, of course, practical.

Many warnings against alternative remedies used for coronavirus have appeared in the media. The mantra is repeated over and over that they are "unproven." That means they have not been subjected to the medical "gold standard": the randomized, controlled trial. (That is not true of Vitamin D, which really should be recommended to everyone.) This approach ignores experience and even established pharmacology. Herbs have been used for millennia, and their properties are known and described. Ours is a different paradigm. Our "proof" is experiential and written on the health of our spirits, souls, and bodies. I thank a kind Creator and Mother Nature for these timeless healing agents.

MATTHEW WOOD has been a practicing herbalist for more than thirty-five years. He received an M.S. in herbal medicine from the Scottish School of Herbal Medicine, accredited by the University of Wales. He is the author of eight books on herbal medicine and a well-known lecturer in the field, now online at Matthew Wood Institute of Herbalism.

NOTES

1. Stephen Harrod Buhner, "Plant-Based Interventions for Coronavirus (SARS-COV-2)," *Stephen Harrod Buhner* (blog), May 17, 2020, stephenharrodbuhner.com/wp-content/uploads/2020/05/coronavirus-1.pdf.

2. A Bruce Boraas, "The better the elimination the better the interior," March 31, 2020, comment on Matthew Wood, "My updated report. Very long," https://www.facebook.com/matthew.wood.5891004/posts/2820096798059618/.

3. "Diagnosis and Treatment of Pneumonitis with a New Coronavirus Infection," compiled by Greta Young Jie De, translated by Jen Ciccolella, website of Pearls of Wisdom Chinese Medicine, March 27, 2020, https://pearlschinesemedicine.com/pow_articles/diagnosis-and-treatment-of-pneumonitis-with-a-new-coronavirus-infection-trial-version-4-compiled-and-translated-by-dr-greta-young-jie-de-ph-d/.

4. Liu Lihong, "Report from the Front Line in Wuhan," translated by Heiner Fruehauf, *Classical Chinese Medicine,* May 8, 2020, http://classicalchinese-medicine.org/report-from-front-line-wuhan.

5. Chen Juan, Huang Di, Wang Shi Qi, and Cai Xiang, "Medical Records from a Young and Brave Female Traditional Chinese Medicine (TCM) doctor on Fighting the COVID-19," pt. 3, compiled and translated by John Chen, eLotus, March 11, 2020, https://www.elotus.org/article/medical-records-young-and-brave-female-traditional-chinese-medicine-tcm-doctor-fighting-covi.

6. NawlinsAg, "Clinical Pearls Covid-19 for ER practitioners," TexAgs forum, March 26, 2020, https://texags.com/forums/84/topics/3102444.

7. "Covid 19-Observations and Plant Medicine Notes, © Judy Lieblein 4/4/2020," PDF. Another herbalist with extensive experience is Michael Cottingham, with whom I corresponded early in the pandemic. We saw eye-to-eye on the herbs necessary for this pandemic. "Matthew Wood," Facebook page, March 2020.

8. Cassandra Willyard, "Corona blood clot mystery intensifies," *Nature,* May 8, 2020, https://www.nature.com/articles/d41586-020-01403-8.

9. "Blood thinners being used to mitigate risk of clots in COVID-19 Patients," *CBS News,* May 26, 2020; https://www.cbsnews.com/news/coronavirus-blood-clots-covid-19-symptom-strokes-young-people.

10. Christen A. Johnson, "Placentas in COVID-positive pregnant women show

injury with blood circulation and clotting," *Chicago Tribune,* May 22, 2020; https://www.chicagotribune.com/coronavirus/ct-life-coronavirus-pregnant -women-placenta-injury-tt-0522-20200522-znymzx45arg6bb2nnpva6tsrz4 -story.html.

11. Will Pass, "Coronavirus Updates: Patients with Covid-19 may face risk of liver injury," *MDedge News,* March 19, 2020, https://www.mdedge.com /chestphysician/article/219309/coronavirus-updates/patients-covid-19 -may-face-risk-liver-injury.

12. NawlinsAg, "Clinical Pearls."

13. Ashley Collman, "CNN anchor Chris Cuomo says the coronavirus has made him lose 13 pounds in 3 days, hallucinate his dead father, and chip a tooth from the chills," *Business Insider,* April 3, 2020, https://www.businessinsider .com/chris-cuomo-coronavirus-lost-13-pounds-2020-4.

14. Rebecca Renner, "The pandemic is giving people vivid, unusual dreams. Here is why," *National Geographic,* April 15, 2020, https://www .nationalgeographic.com/science/2020/04/coronavirus-pandemic-is-giving -people-vivid-unusual-dreams-here-is-why.

15. Email message to author, March 30, 2020.

16. Peter Jackson-Main, "The Sherpas in Nepal apparently use garlic to enable oxygen absorption at high altitude," commenting on Matthew Wood, Facebook page, March 2020.

17. John J Cannell, Michael Zasloff, Cedric F Garland, Robert Scragg, and Edward Giovannucci, "On the epidemiology of influenza," *Virology Journal* 5, no. 29 (February 25, 2008), https://link.springer.com/article /10.1186/1743-422X-5-29.

18. Scott A Read, Stephanie Obeid, Chantelle Ahlenstiel, and Golo Ahlenstiel, "The Role of Zinc in Antiviral Immunity," *Adv Nutr.* 10, no. 4 (July 2019): 696–710, https://www.ncbi.nlm.nih.gov/pmc/articles/PMC6628855/.

19. R. Derwanda and M. Scholz, "Does zinc supplementation enhance the clinical efficacy of chloroquine/hydroxychloroquine to win today's battle against COVID-19?" *Med Hypothesis* 142, no. 109815 (September 2020), https://www.ncbi.nlm.nih.gov/pmc/articles/PMC7202847/.

20. Email message to author, June 22, 2020.

21. Himani Chandna, "Modi govt again advises homoeopathy for COVID-19, suggests sipping water boiled with tulsi," *The Print,* March 18, 2020, https://theprint.in/health/modi-govt-again-advises-homoeopathy-for-covid -19-suggests-sipping-water-boiled-with-tulsi/383363/.

22. Julia Graves, "Flower Essences and Coronavirus," *Green Tara Flower Essences* (blog), http://lilycircle.com/flower-essences-and-coronavirus/.

23. Personal communication with author, March 30, 2020.

24. Centers for Disease Control and Prevention, "What to Do If You Are Sick," website of CDC, May 8, 2020, https://www.cdc.gov/coronavirus/2019-ncov /if-you-are-sick/steps-when-sick.html.

25. Hilda Vargas-Robles, Karla Fabiola Castro-Ochoa, Alí Francisco Citalán-Madrid, and Michael Schnoor, "Beneficial effects of nutritional supplements on intestinal epithelial barrier functions in experimental colitis models *in vivo*," *World J Gastroenterol* 25, no. 30 (August 14, 2019): 4181–98, https://pubmed.ncbi.nlm.nih.gov/31435172/.

26. James M. May and Fiona E. Harrison, "Role of Vitamin C in the Function of the Vascular Endothelium," *Antioxid Redox Signal* 19, no. 17 (December 10, 2013): 2068–83, https://www.ncbi.nlm.nih.gov/pmc/articles /PMC3869438/.

27. Matthew Wood and Phyllis D. Light, "Respiratory System and Respiratory Immunity," website of Matthew Wood Institute of Herbalism, March 28, 2020, https://www.matthewwoodinstituteofherbalism.com/courses /respiratory-system-and-respiratory-immunity.

28. Young Jie De, "Diagnosis and Treatment of Pneumonitis."

29. Young Jie De, "Diagnosis and Treatment of Pneumonitis."

30. Young Jie De, "Diagnosis and Treatment of Pneumonitis."

31. Young Jie De, "Diagnosis and Treatment of Pneumonitis."

32. "Science & Health" section, May 17, 2020; "An Unpredictable Evolution."

33. Yanqing Ding, Huijun Wang, Hong Shen et al., "The Clinical Pathology of Severe Acute Respiratory Syndrome (SARS): A Report From China," *J Pathol* 200, no. 3 (July 2003): 282–89, https://pubmed.ncbi.nlm.nih.gov /12845623/.

34. Young Jie De, "Diagnosis and Treatment of Pneumonitis."

35. Email message to author, March 30, 2020.

36. Email message to author, April 4, 2020.

37. Chandna, "Modi govt again advises homoeopathy."

38. Sen Jo et al., "Characteristics of flavonoids as potent MERS-CoV 3C-like protease inhibitors," *Chemical Biology & Drug Design* 94, no. 6 (Aug 22, 2019): 2023–30, https://onlinelibrary.wiley.com/doi/full/10.1111/cbdd .13604.

39. Email message to author, April 8, 2020.

40. Phyllis Light, "Using a combination of Bayberry, Yarrow, and Cayenne," May 2020, comment on Matthew Wood, Facebook page.

41. "Spiritual Implications of Coronavirus," Facebook group.

42. Ashley Louszko, Knez Walker, Deborah Kim, and Ashley Riegle, "Promises of hope during coronavirus pandemic as people who fell seriously ill begin recovery," *ABC News,* April 3, 2020, https://abcnews.go.com /US/promises-hope-coronavirus-pandemic-people-fell-ill-begin/story?id =69966152.

43. Yeshun Wu et al., "Nervous system involvement after infection with COVID-19 and other coronaviruses," *Brain Behav Immun* 87, (July 2020): 18–22, www.ncbi.nlm.nih.gov/pmc/articles/PMC7146689/.

44. Facebook direct message to author, May 22, 2020.

45. Mohamed Labib Saleh, "Immunomodulaty and therapeutic properties of the *Nigella sativa* L. seed," *Int Immunopharmacol* 5, no. 13-14 (December 2005): 1749–70, https://pubmed.ncbi.nlm.nih.gov/16275613/.

46. Lihong, "Report from the Front Line."

47. "Spiritual Implications of Coronavirus," April 2020.

48. Phyllis Light and William LeSassier, personal communication with author.

49. "Spiritual Implications of Coronavirus," March 2020.

50. Seán Pádraig O'Donoghue, personal communication with author.

51. Seán Pádraig O'Donoghue and others, comment on Matthew Wood, Facebook page, March 2020.

52. Markian Hawryluk, "Heart Damage in COVID-19 Patients Puzzles Doctors," *Scientific American,* April 6, 2020, https://www.scientificamerican.com /article/heart-damage-in-covid-19-patients-puzzles-doctors/.

53. "Spiritual Implications of Coronavirus," March 2020.

54. "Spiritual Implications of Coronavirus," March 2020.

55. Karyn Sanders, personal communication with author.

56. Amanda Dilday, "American Holly ~ What Love Is and What Love Is Not," December 9, 2019, episode 46 in *Whispers: Plant Spirit Medicine,* podcast, https://anchor.fm/amanda-dilday/episodes/Episode-46-American -Holly--What-Love-Is-and-What-Love-Is-Not-e9e3o7.

57. Jinyang Gu, Bing Han, and Jian Wang, "COVID-19: Gastrointestinal Manifestations and Potential Fecal–Oral Transmission," *Gastroenterology* 158, no. 6 (May 1, 2020): 1518–19, https://www.gastrojournal.org/article /S0016-5085(20)30281-X/fulltext

58. Fei Xiao et al., "Evidence for Gastrointestinal Infection of SARS-CoV-2,"

Gastroenterology 158, no. 6 (May 1, 2020): 1831–33, https://www
.gastrojournal.org/article/S0016-5085(20)30282-1/fulltext/.

59. Marcia Frellick, "See acute hepatitis? Consider COVID-19, N.Y. case
suggests," *The Hospitalist,* April 9, 2020, https://www.the-hospitalist
.org/hospitalist/article/220524/coronavirus-updates/see-acute-hepatitis
-consider-covid-19-ny-case?channel=63993/.

60. "Spiritual Implications of Coronavirus," March 2020.

61. Sara Annon, "Coronavirus Issues," PDF (April 2020).

62. "Covid 19-Observations and Plant Medicine Notes," PDF, ©Judy Lieblein
4/4/2020.

63. Jessie Belden, as The Medicine Tree Herbal Pharmacy, comment on
Matthew Wood, Facebook page, March 2020.

64. Katie Walsh, phone call with author, April 5, 2020.

SARS-COV-2
PROTECTION PROTOCOL

Building the Terrain

GABRIEL COUSENS

Let's use this pandemic situation to improve our overall health habits and well-being by observing practices connected to the following broad recommendations and making them more integral parts of our lives:

- Deepening our connection with God
- Engaging in meditation and prayer
- Getting enough sleep (at least 7–8 hours each night)
- Minimizing stress
- Staying hydrated
- Associating with loving people
- Exercising moderately
- Doing breathing exercises every day (*pranayama*) to strengthen lung life force
- Eating an immune-boosting 80 percent raw diet and eating 100 percent vegan
- Utilizing my SARS-CoV-2 Protection Protocol (The location, Wuhan, China, is important because the lethality of the virus, epidemiologically, is increased by 5G and air pollution. The significance

of the word *Wuhan* is that the virus pandemic in Wuhan activated a few weeks after Wuhan turned on its 5G system. Additionally, Wuhan is particularly noted as being high in air pollution.)

The healthier you are and the more proactive steps you take, the more you minimize your chances of catching and/or dying from the coronavirus.

TO PROTECT AND ENHANCE NATURAL IMMUNITY: SARS-COV-2 PROTECTION PROTOCOL

Top Supplements Recommended as Antiviral Protectors

Illumodine—Start with 1 drop in a glass of water 3 times daily. Add one drop to each glass of water each day. Work up to consuming 20 drops in a glass of water 3 times daily (15 minutes or more away from food). Iodine has been shown to destroy SARS and MRSA viruses, and in its atomic form, Illumodine, is probably the most powerful antiviral on the planet.

Nano Silver—1 teaspoon twice daily. Nano Silver has been shown to destroy SARS and MRSA viruses.

Red Algae—2 capsules twice daily such as on waking and bedtime (away from food). Red algae is extremely antiviral.

Zinc—It has been shown through hundreds of studies that zinc supports, rebuilds, and maintains many levels of the immune system. It blocks viral replication. Zinc protects the cell wall from viral invasion and also protects the mitochondria from being invaded by the virus and being used for replicating the virus.

Mega Defense—4 capsules twice daily (for building and protecting the immune system).

Antioxidant Extreme—2 capsules twice daily.

Licorice Root—take as tea or tincture once daily (for lung protection).

Vitamin D—2,000 IU daily (for building the immune system), which has been shown to decrease respiratory infections by 40 percent–50 percent.

Vitamin A—25,000 IU daily (for protecting upper respiratory mucous membranes and lining).

Vitamin C complex—As much as you can take before developing diarrhea.

Two Essential-Oil Blends Recommended for Flying or Traveling

Immortal Immune—to put on the tops of your feet before bed and upon waking (available only at DrCousensOnlineStore.com).

Germs-Be-Gone—to spray on surfaces (such as airplane seats and tables) (available only at DrCousensOnlineStore.com).

Recommended Potential Homeopathics (need to be individualized if infected)

Bryonia

Gelsemium

Eupatorium

Influenzinum 200c to 1M

Tuberculinum 200c to 1M

INCLUDE THESE PROTECTIVE HERBS AND FOODS IN YOUR DIET

The virus enters the cell via a vesicle called an endosome. Once inside, it releases its RNA into the cell cytoplasm and hijacks the cell machinery to produce more viral proteins and thus virus. It also releases an enzyme called 3CL (3-chymotrypsin-like protease). This enzyme attacks and weakens the cell's defense mechanism against these coronavirus attack molecules.

These suggested herbal remedies destroy the coronavirus 3CL

enzyme and thus preserve the cell's ability to protect itself. The best nutraceuticals for destroying the 3CL enzyme are **quercetin** and **epigallocatechin gallate,** which is found in **green tea** and **green tea extract**. These anti-3CL substances are also found in:

flax seed

citrus peel

tickberry leaves

orange peel

oregano

garlic

ginger

elderberry

turmeric

ESSENTIAL OILS TO PROTECT FROM SARS-COV-2

You can apply small amounts of essential oil on tops of feet, wrists, and chest (as well as to your face mask). Diluting with a carrier oil is recommended for sensitive skin. The most important essential oils, which were key for prevention and healing during the bubonic plague and perhaps now, are the following:

eucalyptus

clove

grapefruit

cinnamon

tea tree

lemon grass

frankincense

oregano

Immortal Immune—rub on tops of feet twice daily

Germs-Be-Gone—spray on all surfaces you may touch and also on
   any face mask you wear. Also spray on hands and rub on when-

ever you have to touch potentially contaminated surfaces like cash or on public transportation.

Add some of the above essential oils and supplements to your overall prevention system. ***The key concept is prevention.***

At whatever level things are happening, the world has already changed in a major way. If we approach this crisis with love, compassion, and thoughtfulness, rather than fear, we have the opportunity to expand the global consciousness to a new level of positive awareness. We could be in the birth pangs of the creation of a New Heaven and New Earth. This is an opportunity to go within to focus on one's meaning and life purpose—and in this waking-up process, return to God.

The best defense is always a good offense, which is to build and strengthen every level of one's "terrain" (your general protective life-force energy and immune system) with a full holistic lifestyle upgrade. We now have a great reason, imminent opportunity, or at least a good excuse to do this. Maintain a dedicated level of this protocol composed of antiviral and immunity-building supplements and nutrients and observe good personal antiviral hygiene. As the Sufis say, "Love everyone, and tie up your camel." By following this approach there's no need to go into fear, as fear undermines the immune system. Being at peace and in a state of love builds the immune system.

We have choices, and may we be blessed to make the choices that protect ourselves, our families, and the ethical, moral, and spiritual health of our local and world society and Global Brain. And in this process may we be blessed to be able to uplift the planetary consciousness and love of humanity.

BLESSINGS TO YOUR HEALTH, WELL-BEING, AND SPIRIT.
—RABBI GABRIEL COUSENS, M.D., M.D.(H.), N.D.(H.C.), D.D.,
DIP. AMERICAN BOARD OF HOLISTIC INTEGRATIVE MEDICINE,
DIP. AYURVEDA

GABRIEL COUSENS is a holistic orthomolecular physician, homeopath, psychiatrist, family therapist, Ayurvedic practitioner, Chinese herbalist, and ordained rabbi. He has served as a lieutenant commander in the U.S. Public Health Service and is a former member of the board of trustees of the American Board of Holistic Integrative Medicine and is currently vice president of the Arizona Board of Holistic Integrative Medicine (AHIMA).

COVID-19 PROTOCOL

Jus Crea Giammarino

RECOMMENDED IMMUNE SUPPORT: THE BASICS

Do not eat sugar, dairy, white flour. Avoid alcohol and smoking. Avoid processed foods and chemically grown foods, i.e., with pesticides that kill off the microbiome, as this is vital for immune function. Feed beneficial flora with lacto-fermented foods such as miso, kimchee, etc. Avoid any food sensitivities or intolerances that increase inflammation.

Eat an organic whole-foods diet with lots of nutrient-dense fruits, veggies, beans, nuts/seeds, meats, fish, and whole grains.

Immune-boosting foods include sage, rosemary, thyme, oregano (very powerful), turmeric, garlic, ginger, onion, leeks, Fire cider, Four Thieves vinegar, and lacto-fermented foods such as miso and kimchee.

Drink herbal teas. Immune-boosting teas can be made from white pine, chaga (a medicinal mushroom), balsam fir bark or needles, astragalus. Make bone and/or veggie broths. Broth is excellent, especially if you eat the marrow after it is done boiling (homemade is best).

Get adequate sleep and rest.

Get outdoors for sunshine, exercise, fresh air, and forest bathing. Yoga, relaxation, meditation, garden, gratitude, prayer, connection, nature.

Practice good hygiene and "social distancing."

Use soap. Do not use Lysol or other carcinogens. Avoid triclosan in hand sanitizers. Use thyme, eucalyptus, and other antimicrobial essential oils for room sprays and diffusers.

PREVENTIVE HERBS AND SUPPLEMENTS— IMMUNE BUILDING

Many of these herbal medicines are regionally specific for Penobscot and Abenaki in Maine but are widely known by herbalists.

Elderberry syrup or tincture

Echinacea

Reishi, turkey tail, and chaga teas or tinctures

Flagroot or bear root tea or just chew on it. Can also wear it as protection. Carry it in medicine pouch.

If you get the virus, eliminate elderberry and echinacea and don't take Advil—everything else is still good for you.**

Get adequate rest and sound sleep.

VITAMIN SUPPORT

Vitamin A: 5,000–25,000 IU/day; carotenoids, carrots, pumpkin, squash

Vitamin C: 1000 mg–bowel tolerance; try high-dose Vitamin C pure powder (Solaray has a 4500mg powder)

Vitamin D3: 2000–10,000 IU/day

Zinc: lots of zinc in pumpkin seeds or take a zinc lozenge 2–3 times a day (5–50,000mg/day)

NAC: 500–1500/day to prevent lung fibrosis

Probiotics: 25–75 billion/day

I also swear by Wellness Formula by Source Naturals.

FOR ANXIETY

Rescue Remedy, GABA, l-theanine or herbal formula

Nervines: wild milky oat, skullcap (an endangered native species), among many others.

Lemon balm tea or tincture 2–3 times a day helps with anxiety and is also good for the immune system generally. It's an antiviral herb.

Adaptogens for stress and resiliency, including licorice (also antiviral), ginseng, rhodiola, ashwaganda.

CLEANING

Use Thieves essential oil on your hands, nostrils, and mouth whenever you have to leave the house—better than any hand sanitizer on the market. Don't put it inside your nose, just all around the outside of your nostrils. It will burn a little, but it only lasts a few minutes.

House cleansing: In addition to normal cleaning (with safe natural cleaners), boil cedar on the stove to clear the air and smudge with sage to kill microbes. You can also make a mixture with *Eucalyptus globulus* essential oil and water and spray surfaces—it's a good anti-microbial, anti-viral, anti-bacterial, and anti-fungal. Try diffusing eucalyptus in the home. You can also steam with thyme, pine, cedar, or balsam.

ACTIVE VIRUS PROTOCOL

Use these teas for fever 99–102 degrees: Yarrow and/or Bone Set (for when the fever sets in the bones and gives you body aches), Elder Flowers. Yarrow and Bone Set actually support the fever and allow it to do its work.

Fever over 102 degrees: Add neutral baths and cool compresses. **Hydration!!**

**Fever over 103 degrees: Seek medical assistance.

Difficulty breathing: Seek medical assistance immediately.

LUNG HERBS AND OILS

Mullein leaf (this can also be smoked), coltsfoot, thyme, osha or bear root: You can make tea with all of these. Make a big pot and drink several cups a day. With the bear root/osha you can also chew on a small piece throughout the day.

Usnea and lobelia help breathing. Pleurisy root, grindelia, elecampane are Lung herbs.

Eucalyptus steams: Boil a pot of water. Place boiling water in a bowl. Add 6–7 drops of eucalyptus essential oil (either *Eucalyptus globulus* or *Eucalyptus radiata*), wait one minute (trust me, if not you'll burn your nostrils), then put a towel over your head and the bowl and steam for 10–15 minutes. Do this 2–3 times a day (also good for sinus cold).

Also thyme essential oil is very good antiseptic and steam.

Ravensara essential oil: Just open the bottle and inhale for one minute 3–4 times a day. Great for tonifying the lungs.

Oregano essential oil is a powerful anti-viral (it can get rid of anthrax). You can put two drops of this on the bottom of your feet 2–3 times a day, or mix 1–2 drops with a carrier oil (olive oil is good) and take internally every 4–8 hours.

ACUTE HERBAL FORMULAS

Fever: Boneset, Elderflowers, Yarrow, Catnip

Cough/Lungs: Osha, Elecampane, Mullein, Grindelia, Coltsfoot, Lobelia, Pleurisy root

Antivirals: Licorice, Lomatium, Lemon Balm, Elder, Chaparral, St. John's Wort, Andrographis

Immune supportive: White pine, Cedar, Rose hips, Medicinal mushrooms (Cordyceps, Reishi, Turkey Tail, Chaga)

Anti-inflammatories: Turmeric, Proteolytic enzymes (Serralase or Nattokinase to prevent blood clots)

HOMEOPATHIC FIRST AID KIT

Fever: Bryonia, Eupatorium, Gelsemium, Belladonna
Cough: Spongia, Drosera
Antiviral and upper respiratory: Mucocconinum, V-Clear

HYDROTHERAPY

Wet socks, fever treatment, steam inhalations with essential oils (thyme or eucalyptus)

Thanks to Sherri Mitchell for some of the information in this brief summary.

Raised with her Penobscot culture and Native American spiritual practices, Dr. Jus Crea realized the healing powers of nature at a young age. Rich with ancestral knowledge of healing, medicine, and midwifery, Jus Crea received a doctorate in naturopathic medicine from the University of Bridgeport and a B.S. in ethnobotany and holistic health from UMass, Amherst. She has also been trained as an auricular acupuncture detox specialist at Lincoln Hospital, in WTS therapy for restorative healing, as well as Indigenous midwifery with Mewinzha Ondaadiziike Wiigaming. Dr. Jus Crea has lectured extensively on healing, ethnobotany, midwifery, naturopathic medicine, environmental medicine, and cultural history and traditions. She was previously an adjunct professor of nutrition at Springfield College and Pathology at STCC, as well as a primary care physician in Brattleboro, Vermont. Jus Crea has been practicing naturopathic family medicine at The Integrative Health Group in Springfield, Massachusetts, since RSST. She is passionate about cultural healing practices and works towards reclamation of her Wabanaki traditions, spiritual practices, and language.

HOMEOPATHY, VITAL FORCE, AND CORONA

Vatsala Sperling

INTRODUCTION:
THE VIRUS AS A FORCE OF EVOLUTION

At the moment all of us, from three to one hundred and three years old, have one word on our lips—Virus! What is a virus after all but an entity much smaller than bacteria that lives like an inert molecule of dust until it finds a host? The host—a living cell of bacteria, fungi, plants, animals, or humans—is necessary for a virus to replicate itself and increase its numbers. If it fails to find a host, it can't do much more than spend its days in utter tranquility just like a particle of dust.

However, there is a difference between an inert particle of dust and a virus. Unlike dust, a virus contains within its sturdy coat made of proteins and lipids a supply of genetic material: single strands of ribonucleic acid (RNA), deoxyribonucleic acid (DNA), or both RNA and DNA. In this simple form and structure, viruses have been around since the very first living cells evolved millions of years ago, in many ways serving as the unsung heroes of the ecosystem. They have been helping with the destruction of bacteria and release of the structural components of bacteria back into the ecosystem so that these components are available for use by other living cells.

Viruses play an important role in the landscape of genetic material. Once they find a suitable host, viruses move genetic material horizontally and help increase genetic diversity by transferring genetic material between different species. Viruses are thus the driving force behind evolution. Nature deploys several vectors that act as a bridge between the viruses and their hosts. These vectors could be insects that feed on plants or suck blood from animals. The vector insects acquire a vast supply of virus from one host, and while visiting another host for a meal of plant sap or blood, they donate their collection of viruses to the new host. Some viruses spread via droplets that escape from the oral-nasal route while sneezing, and even talking and spitting. Some other viruses accompany excreta. Flying insects visit the excreta, pick up viruses on their feet and wings, and carry them to food and water. A new host ingests viruses as he consumes the contaminated food and water. Some other viruses spread among hosts via exchange of blood and body fluids.

Once inside the host cell, viruses shed their coat, integrate their genetic material into the genetic material of the host cells, and begin to proliferate. The newly replicated viral genetic strands use the proteins and lipids from the host to assemble new coats. Now fully formed, the viruses are released from the host cells either by lysis (total destruction) of the host cells, or by budding of the host cell. Some types of viruses integrate their genetic material into the host genetic material and do not destroy the host cells. These infected host cells can function normally as the viral genetic material moves vertically from one generation of the cell to the next when the host cell undergoes cell division.

Thousands of species of viruses are known, and many more thousands are yet to be identified and named. Many hundreds of acute and chronic diseases in plants, animals, and humans are attributed to viruses. At least 219 species of viruses are known to infect humans and cause serious illnesses,[1,2,3,4,5] and they are associated with numerous epidemics and pandemics killing millions of people worldwide.[6,7,8,9,10]

The latest pandemic to slash its way across every continent is COVID-19 caused by Corona virus.[11,12,13] However, pandemics are not a new experience for humanity. Over the course of centuries of recorded history of infectious diseases, pandemics have brought humanity face to face with its place in the hierarchy that plays out in the interaction and relationship between species. These waves of disease force humans to ask serious questions about life itself and ponder our powerlessness against invisible infectious agents.[14]

Though the infectious agents have enormous striking power, the human race is a tenacious one. Every time a new pandemic came along and began charting its brutal path through humanity, the society came up with ways and means to check the spread of the infectious disease. As science and technology evolved, vaccines were developed a few years after an outbreak.

TABLE I.
U.S. EPIDEMICS, PANDEMICS, AND VACCINES[15, 16, 17, 18, 19, 20, 21, 22, 23, 24, 25, 26, 27]

Disease/ location	Year/ duration of outbreak	Casualty	Vaccine development
Smallpox from European settlers New England	1633–1634	>70% of Native American population dropped	1770
Yellow fever Philadelphia	1793	5000 people died	1935
Cholera New York City	1832–1866	2–6 Americans died daily	1896
Scarlet fever New England	1858	95% of patients were children	No vaccine available
Typhoid New York area	1906–1907	10,771 deaths	1896

TABLE I.
U.S. EPIDEMICS, PANDEMICS, AND VACCINES (cont.)

Disease/ location	Year/ duration of outbreak	Casualty	Vaccine development
Spanish Flu Entire United States	1918–1920	675,000 Americans died; 17–50 million deaths worldwide	1942
Asian Flu	1957	70,000 Americans died	Because of mutation in Flu virus, new vaccines are needed frequently
Diphtheria Entire United States	1921–1925	15,520 deaths	1925–1926
Polio Entire United States	1916–1955	3,145 deaths	1955
Measles Entire United States	1981–1991 2014–2015	2,000–10,000 deaths annually	1989
Whooping cough California	2010, 2014	10 infants died out of 10,000 cases	1940s
AIDS Chimpanzee is a natural reservoir	1980s to present	675,000 deaths till 2016; 13,000 deaths annually since then	No vaccine available
Bird flu H5N1 Aquatic birds and poultry are reservoirs	2003	High fatality rate, but virus does not spread among people	2007

TABLE I.
U.S. EPIDEMICS, PANDEMICS, AND VACCINES (cont.)

Disease/ location	Year/ duration of outbreak	Casualty	Vaccine development
SARS coronavirus Bats are reservoirs	Early 2003. Spreads quickly. Threat faded in 2004. Spread to 32 countries.	800 deaths	2004, by then the SARS epidemic was over
MERS coronavirus Bats are reservoirs	2012	858 deaths	1st human trial in July 2019
SWINE flu HINI Pigs are reservoirs	2009–2010	150,000– 575,000 deaths worldwide	2009
EBOLA Bats are reservoirs	2013–2016	11,323 deaths as of May 2016	2016
Novel coronavirus COVID-19 aka SARS-CoV-2 Affecting 213 countries Bats and pangolins are reservoirs	End of 2019 till present	25,373,482 cases worldwide, 850,047 deaths as of August 30, 2020.	BABL/c mice have been tested for subcutaneous vaccine using dissolvable microneedle arrays. Vaccines for humans not available yet.

AIDS, Bird flu, SARS, MERS, Swine flu, and the latest COVID-19 or SARS-CoV-2—each one of these outbreaks of epidemics and pandemics has a few common points:

1. There is an animal reservoir that carries the virus but does not show any symptoms of the disease.

2. Humans get infected from hunting, slaughtering, handling, eat-

ing, or living in close proximity with the reservoir species.

3. The virus begins to spread among humans. Some begin to show disease symptoms. Some become carriers/reservoirs and do not show any symptoms. Human-to-human transmission occurs via well-known transmission routes. Direct transmission through blood and body fluids spreads AIDS and other sexually transmitted diseases. Indirect transmission occurs via airborne particles, fomites, droplets, and vectors.

4. In earlier centuries, modes of transportation were slow. Fewer people traveled to foreign countries. Rate of international trade and commerce was slow too. The present century has exactly the opposite scenario. People from every country can (and often do) travel and visit almost any other country. The commercial airlines can bring in thousands of carrier and slightly unwell individuals to a country in just 30 hours, and once they spread out into and mingle with the population of the host country, the disease begins to spread like wildfire. This is what happened with COVID-19. Though the disease began in China, it has spread to every continent.

5. It takes several years of exorbitantly expensive research and development, as well as human trials, before a cost-effective, safe, and reliable vaccine is available for the public. And no vaccine is 100% effective.

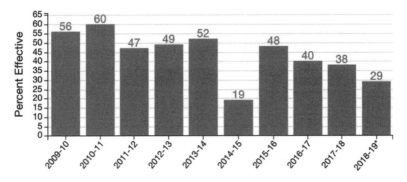

Seasonal Flu Vaccine Effectiveness

6. Particularly with regard to the flu, there is no universal vaccine with 100% effectiveness. Viruses causing flu mutate rapidly, and newer strains emerge against which the vaccines of earlier years are either ineffective or provide protection to less than 60% of those receiving vaccination.[28]

SIMILARITIES AND DIFFERENCES BETWEEN THE FLU AND COVID-19

The novel COVID-19 caused by Coronavirus elicits some symptoms similar to regular flu (caused by Influenza virus), but it has some unique symptoms too. In early stages fever, cough, body aches, fatigue, and occasionally vomiting/diarrhea are common to both. Both spread among people as they release virus-loaded droplets and aerosol while talking, breathing, spitting, coughing, and sneezing. Both illnesses can be spread by asymptomatic carriers and very mildly symptomatic individuals in whom the virus is in the incubation period and the prodromal stage. Both these viruses cannot be treated with antibiotics (antibiotics do work against bacteria but not viruses). At an advanced stage of infection with lung involvement, intensive hospital-based care with mechanical ventilators would be required.[29,30,31]

As shown in the diagram above, various flu vaccines are available with effectiveness between 19 and 60 percent. Since COVID-19 is caused by a new virus, no vaccine is available.

Though COVID-19 is another coronavirus like SARS-CoV (associated with earlier Coronavirus outbreaks), it has different epidemiological characteristics. COVID-19 is very efficient in replicating in the upper respiratory tract and causes a less abrupt onset of symptoms. In the prodromal period, the infected individuals produce large quantities of the virus in their upper respiratory tract, and since they are not quite sick yet, they carry on with their usual daily activities and spread the virus to their contacts. For this reason, it has been quite hard to contain the spread of COVID-19.

COVID-19 causes, like seasonal influenza, mild and self-limiting disease in most people who are infected. Severe illness with pneumonia and lung involvement is caused in older people with co-morbid conditions such as diabetes, hypertension, and other chronic illnesses.

Since no vaccines and coronavirus antivirals are available for COVID-19, non-pharmaceutical interventions are the mainstay in containment of the disease in the community.[32] This includes hand washing, face masks, social distancing, self-isolation, canceling public gatherings, school closures, remote working, home isolation, curfews, quarantine, lockdown, and so on. The level of public education about COVID-19 is very different from what it used to be during earlier outbreaks of Coronavirus and other flu epidemics and pandemics. Now there is 24/7 real and fake news and many platforms of social media that spread information about COVID-19 as fast as your internet connection will allow. And yet, flattening of the COVID-19 curve has remained elusive.

Non-pharmaceutical intervention implies that there is room for alternative approaches.

India has set an example in this regard by proposing the use of a homeopathic remedy. Unfazed by the harsh criticism hurled at it by the mainstream from both India and abroad, the government of India and its ministry AYUSH (Ayurveda, Yoga and Naturopathy, Unani, Siddha, and Homeopathy) recommend the homeopathic remedy Arsenicum album in 30c[33] doses as preventive for COVID-19. This is being used enthusiastically and successfully by the public. The Ministry of AYUSH functions alongside the Ministry of Health and Family welfare (since 2003) and is well aware of the role of Homeopathy in successfully handling epidemics and pandemics in earlier centuries.

TABLE 2. TREATMENT OF EPIDEMICS WITH HOMEOPATHY—A SUCCINCT HISTORY[34]

Epidemic	Year	Mortality in conventional treatment	Mortality in cases treated with Homeopathy
Scarlet fever Germany	1799	—	<5%
Typhus fever Ireland, England	1813	30%	180 cases treated by Samuel Hahnemann; 2 deaths
Cholera Russia, Europe	1830–1892	40%–80%	Hahnemann developed the idea of genus epidemicus; 7–9%
Yellow fever USA	1850s	15–85%	5–6.7%
Pneumonia Austria	Mid 1800s	20%	5%
Diphtheria	1862–1864	83.6 %	16.4%
Spanish flu pandemic	1918	28.2%	<1%–1.05%
Polio	1950s	Prophylactic treatment of a few thousand cases; not one developed polio	

Scientists, medical doctors, and homeopaths from Finlay Institute, Cuba, have been using homeo-prophylaxis for seasonal epidemics like leptospirosis.[35]

HISTORY OF HOMEOPATHY IN INDIA

During British rule, Homeopathy was brought to India in 1839 by a Romanian homeopath, John Honigberger, who was a direct disciple of Samuel Hahnemann, M.D. (1755–1843, the founder of Homeopathy).

Since then India has a proven track record of its relationship with Homeopathy. This country is fertile ground for a holistic and low-cost medical system like Homeopathy. The very first medical college of Homeopathy was founded in Calcutta in 1881, then the capital of British India. In 1973, Homeopathy was recognized as a national system of medicine, and the Central Council of Homeopathy was established to oversee and regulate the education and practice of Homeopathy. Presently, Homeopathy is the third most popular system of medical treatment after Allopathy (mainstream Western medicine) and Ayurveda (a comprehensive medical specialty that originated in India many thousands of years ago). There are over 195 medical colleges, more than 200,000 registered practitioners with government-recognized homeopathic medical degrees, and 38 postgraduate colleges offering an M.D. degree in Homeopathy, with 12,000 new graduates added to the pool every year.[36,37,38]

Homeopathy education funded, encouraged, and supported by taxpayer money, together with legal recognition and protection provided by the democratically elected government, translates into absence of fear and suppression around Homeopathy education and practice and use of this modality by the public, as evidenced by a 25 percent annual growth rate of Homeopathy in India. It is not surprising that the latest research and advancement in Homeopathy comes from India.[39,40,41,42]

Because of easy access to homeopathic education, research, and remedies, and also because of multi-generational uninterrupted use of Homeopathy for common and serious illness, it is common knowledge among the population in India that homeopathic remedies do not have any side effects and are safe for all age groups including pregnant women and newborn babies. Homeopathy is thus woven into the very fabric of India and is available in every town and village. About 10 percent of the population relies on Homeopathy for its complete health care.

COVID-19: BRING IT ON, WE CAN HANDLE IT!

Reading what the leading homeopaths from India have to say about how to deal with COVID-19 offers hope and confidence in the face of this novel threat to the health and well-being of humanity.

In a recent interview Dr. Ajit Kulkarni pointed out that addressing epidemics and pandemics is nothing new in Homeopathy, which has an extensive track record of successfully reducing morbidity and mortality during outbreaks of infectious diseases.[43] The Government of India has based its decision to use Homeopathy during the current COVID-19 outbreak on the available record of Homeopathy's efficacy in handling epidemics and pandemics.

Dr. Kulkarni explained a day-by-day progression of COVID-19 symptoms:

People infected with the COVID-19 can remain symptom-free for anywhere from 14 to 27 days. During this time, the virus is replicating in their upper respiratory tract and escapes into the surroundings via droplets that are released during coughing, sneezing, speaking, etc. These droplets are inhaled by those nearby. The virus-loaded droplets land on fomites (objects and materials likely to carry infection such as clothing) and other inanimate surfaces, where the virus can remain viable for several days. Once symptoms begin to appear, progression is more or less as given below:

Days 1–3:

Cold and flu-like symptoms

Fever

Mild or no throat pain

Day 4:

Increased soreness and pain in throat

Fever between 97 and 98 degrees Fahrenheit

Mild headache

Diarrhea and cramps

Day 5:

Throat pain very severe, worse from eating and drinking

Voice is affected

Dry cough sets in

Joint pains are worse on moving

Weakness

Day 6:

Fever rises to 98.6 degrees F

Symptoms of days 1–5 increase in intensity

Nausea, vomiting, and diarrhea

Mild feeling of shortness of breath

Body aches and pains from joints to fingers

Increase in weakness

Day 7:

Fever rises to 100.4 degrees F

Excessive cough

All above symptoms get worse

Day 8:

Excessive dry cough

Severe difficulty breathing

Heaviness and pain in chest

Toxic and ill appearance with intense weakness

Fever above 100.4 degrees

Day 9:

All symptoms much worse

Cyanosis

Kidney failure

Respiratory failure

Multi-organ failure

All patients do not follow and present a pattern of illness exactly as mentioned above. However, the typical day-by-day progression of the disease is very useful information that helps the homeopaths in choosing a suitable remedy and managing the disease.

Based on his observation of the evolution and totality of symptoms, Kulkarni has proposed a treatment plan.

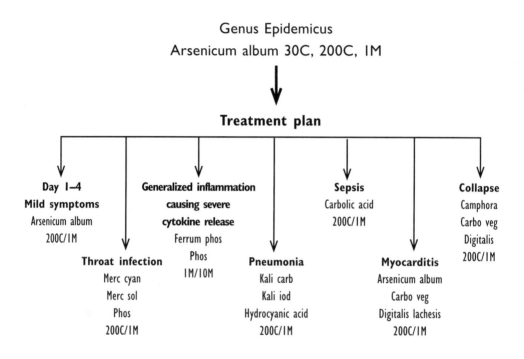

Kulkarni cautions that even though many remedies can be considered for treatment of COVID-19, any chosen remedy must augment the immune response against inhibition of viral replication, promote viral clearance, induce tissue repair, and trigger the adaptive mechanisms. From a homeopathic perspective, Kulkarni reiterates that the practitioners must adhere to the fundamentals of case taking with particular emphasis on location, sensation, and pathology, modalities as well as concomitants. At every instance, the practitioner must understand the stage where the patient is and apply the Law of Similars for selecting the remedy.

To illustrate how the symptom picture matches the remedy picture: take, for example, the symptoms that appear during critical stage when the patient seems to be on his deathbed gasping for breath. He is showing cyanosis from lack of oxygen, his blood oxygen level is low, he shows air-hunger. His lungs and heart are failing. Lung is filled up with debris and pus. He is in shock. At this time, administering Carbo vegetabilis brings him back and his symptoms can be reversed.

Kulkarni suggests that remedies can be repeated frequently as needed.

TABLE 3. KULKARNI'S RECOMMENDATIONS FOR COVID-19 AND PNEUMONIAS

Severity of case	Recommended remedies
Mild to moderate	Arsenicum album, Bryonia alba, Chelidonium, Eupatoreum perfoliatum, Ferrum phosphoricum, Gelsemium, Hepar sulphuris calcareum, Mercurius solubilis, and Mercurius cyanatus
Severe cases	Apis mellifica, Arsenicum album, Bryonia, Camphora, Kali carbonicum, Kali iodatum, Lycopodium, Phosphorus, Pyrogenium, Sulphur, and Tuberculinum
Critical cases	Arsenicum album, Antimonium tartaricum, Camphora, Carbolicum acidicum, Carbo vegetabilis, Carbo animalis, Hippozenium, Kali carbonicum, Kali iodatum, Sulphur, and Veratrum album
Incipient pneumonias*	Aconitum, Belladonna, Ferrum phosphoricum, and Ipecaccuanha
Frankly developed pneumonias *	Bryonia, Phosphorus, Veratrum viridae, and Chelidonium. For complicated pneumonias, Baptisia, Pyrogenium, Lachesis, Mercurius solubilis, Hepar sulphuris calcareum, and Rhus toxicodendron
Complicated pneumonias*	Baptisia, Pyrogenium, Lachesis, Mercurius solubilis, Hepar sulphuris calcareum, and Rhus toxicodendron
Definite bronchopneumonia*	Natrum sulphuricum, Pulsatilla, Senega, Lobelia inflata
Late pneumonias *	Antimonium tartaricum, Carbo vegetabilis, Kali carbonicum, Lycopodium, Arsenicum album, and Sulphur, Ferrum phosphoricum in 1m, 10m

*Kulkarni has based the grading of pneumonias and his choice of remedies on the classic work of Douglas M. Borland, *Pneumonias*, first published in 1939 in the UK.[44]

From Italy, Massimo Mangialavori reported working with eighty-four patients.[45] He used Chininum muriaticum for those with fever resistant to common antipyretics, rising in the early afternoon, weakness more pronounced in the evenings, frontal headache with painful pressure and intense eye pain, dry cough perceived as discomfort in the upper respiratory tract, poor appetite, and little thirst.

Mangialavori also used Grindelia robusta for these symptoms: fever with sudden increase in temperature, weakness more evident in early morning, throbbing headache in the occiput, better by sitting, with a desire to lie down but pain does not allow them to lie down, dry cough with desire to expectorate but absence of phlegm, struggles to get rid of the small amount of mucus, paroxysms of suffocating cough, anxiety with breathing difficulty, and a feeling that he must quickly go to a hospital, worried about falling asleep and not being able to breathe during sleep, wants to sleep with a light on, conjunctivitis moving from one eye to the other, joint pain in lower limbs, fearful, aware of being worried about symptoms.

Mangialavori also used Cinnamomum camphora for the following symptoms that he observed in his patients: continuous fever, sweating, chills, incipient fatigue worsening with sweating, headache with pressure from inside, wants to find relief by binding head tightly, cough less than the two previous remedies but tiring nevertheless, deep inhalation brings on cough. Shallow breathing seems to bring in insufficient amount of oxygen. Worry leads to more deep breathing and more cough. Shortness of breath from minimal exertion, watery and persistent post-nasal drip, diarrhea without abdominal pain, scanty urine, feels confused about being dangerous to one's family members.

With use of the three remedies for indicated symptoms, 64 of 84 patients overcame their symptoms in more or less 3–4 days. They declared clear improvement and reported no relapse.

Dr. Manish Bhatia has done an extensive study of all the available and published COVID-19 symptoms.[46] He observes that in Wuhan, Iran, and Italy, the disease has been very severe with patients complaining of respiratory distress and collapse. In other parts of the world, disease seems to be milder. In India, for example, a large number of patients seem to be asymptomatic or are developing very mild symptoms. He has compared the mortality rate of COVID-19 with other flus encountered in recent times and concluded that COVID-19 is not a life-threatening infection for most people. His observation is supported by recent reports from Santa Clara, California.[47] Children and young adults just get flu-like symptoms, and maximum mortality rate is seen in elderly with pre-existing health complications. A similar comparison is available from other sources as well.[48]

Infection/epidemic	Mortality
Ebola	50–90%
H5N1 Bird flu	50%
SARS	15%
Dengue	1%
H1N1 Swine flu	0.02%
Measles	0.2%
Seasonal flu	0.1%
Spanish flu	2%
COVID-19	0.4–3.4%

In his study, Bhatia found that remedies such as Bryonia, Lycopodium, Mercurius solubilis, and Kali carbonicum cover the laterality, sequence, and pace of symptoms of COVID-19 infection. He recommends Bryonia as a prophylactic too and in low potency; it can be taken daily where cases of COVID-19 infection are clustered. Bryonia also covers the seasonality, as hemispheres transition from winter to spring with nights cold and days warm. Bryonia covers the respiratory symptoms of COVID-19 very well: cough dry, hard, very painful, at night, as from stomach, must sit up, worse from eating, drinking, wants to take deep breath but cannot as it excites cough; expectoration rusty, blood-streaked or tough; bronchitis, asthma, pneumonia, sharp stitches in chest or at right scapula, worse deep breathing and coughing, pleurisy, coming to warm room excites cough, holds chest, presses at sternum when coughing.

Similarly, Lycopodium and Kali carb cover the symptoms of COVID-19 infection. A detailed description of symptoms of these remedies can be found in textbooks of Homeopathy written over a century ago.[49]

Drs. Rajan Sankaran and Aditya Kasariyans analyzed the symptom presentation of 30 COVID-19 cases (40–70 years old) in Iran, and for 26 out of 30 patients, they prescribed Camphora 1M. [50,51] A few other patients were given Arsenicum album, China, and Phosphorus depending on the totality of their symptoms. The cases had either positive lab test / Corona test or positive CT scan. Patients receiving Camphora were at different stages of the disease. Some had just started having symptoms, some were very sick, and some others had several different complications. Without exception, they showed a dramatic response to Camphora by overcoming extreme prostration, low energy, and nausea. Body aches, soreness, breathlessness, and cough reduced within 24 hours. Their health improved significantly, and Oxygen saturation increased. Symptoms improved by 40 percent within 24–30 hours of the first prescription, and morbidity was reduced significantly.

Drs. Sachindra and Bhawisha Joshi have proposed use of Bryonia alba, Arsenicum album, and Phosphorus for early/mild cases and Antimonium tartaricum, Grindelia, and Camphora for severe symptoms with breathlessness and low oxygen.[52]

In an integrated approach, Dr. Dinesh Chauhan has made the following recommendations:[53]

1. Lobelia purpurascens: Profound prostration, respiratory paralysis, deadly chills without shivering, influenza, oppression of lower parts of chest.
2. Quebracho: Low oxygen (it can be considered a homeopathic oxygen mask).
3. Grindelia: Asthma, emphysema, smothering suffocation on falling asleep, desire for light, sunshine, and company.

4. Quillaja saponaria: Colds with dry sore throat, cough with difficult expectoration. Quillaja Saponaria is a homeopathic remedy that uses the medicinal properties of the saponin content of the plant. Saponins are known to have an antiviral action. Now, it is interesting that handwashing for 20 seconds with soap (a derivative of saponin) and warm water has been recommended for prevention of COVID-19. Both soap and warm water destroy the integrity of the viral lipid coat.

Dr. Chauhan further recommends Bach flower essences, herbal teas, as well as books to read during the lockdowns so that our knowledge may increase.

Working from the east of India in Calcutta, one of the most crowded cities of the world, and with five generations of homeopaths in the family, Dr. Saparishi Banerjea recommends the remedies Sticta pulmonaria, Justicia adhatoda, Spongia toasta, Bryonia alba, Rumex crispus, Rhus toxicodendron, Eucalyptus, Ferrum phosphoricum, Arsenicum album, and Gelsemium.[54] Similarly, the work of Harry Van Der Jee[55] gives a deep insight into the current COVID-19 pandemic and helps make sense of it. From Mumbai, India, Dr. Divya Chabbra offers her remedy suggestions for dealing with COVID-19 infection.[56]

AS MANY HOMEOPATHS, THAT MANY REMEDIES: WHAT TO CHOOSE, HOW TO TAKE REMEDIES?

With so many different recommendations from various homeopaths, choosing a suitable remedy might seem to be a daunting task, and rightly so. But what is necessary to remember here is that COVID-19 symptoms have not been constant throughout the world. There have been asymptomatic carriers. There have been mildly sick individuals. Some have become extremely sick and required ventilators. Some of those have returned home after recovery but many of them have died.

What is apparent from the work of homeopaths from India is that for every stage of the disease, several homeopathic remedies are available. When chosen with particular attention to the symptoms of the patient, the remedies cut short the morbidity and arrest the progression of the disease.

It is a known factor in infectious diseases that an individual's susceptibility plays a very strong role in how he or she will manifest symptoms. Some people live through epidemics and pandemics, some others die. Some recover from illness, some show no signs and symptoms of the disease. These differences in the outcome raise a question—why some of us are susceptible to infectious disease whereas others get the same microbe and remain well. For most of human history, it was believed to be luck. Upon their discovery by scientists, germs became the favorite punching bag and villains that brought on infectious diseases (and with invention of antibiotics, the public was led to believe that we will live in a world free from infectious diseases). But these assumptions do not explain the varying outcome and expression in different individuals when they get the same germ. Examining susceptibility in the context of "damage-response framework" helps us understand the several factors that influence the outcome of an individual's interaction with an infectious agent.

1. Microbe: Virulence, inoculum, pathogenicity
2. Host: Sex, age, nutrition, immunity, history, exposure, chance, genetics
3. Environment: Temperature, humidity, population density, hygiene, climate, presence of environmental toxins

With all these factors playing a role together, it is incorrect to expect that every single person exposed to a pathogen will develop exactly the same symptoms.[57]

However, the overall expression of symptoms during an epidemic and pandemic does have a common pattern of presentation, as if the community is responding as one entity to infection by a pathogen. This idea formed the basis of Dr. Samuel Hahnemann's choice of a homeopathic remedy as genus epidemicus for the various epidemics that he treated in his lifetime and obtained stellar results.[58] In treating the epidemics of his time, Hahnemann considered the general, generic symptoms of the epidemic displayed by all patients instead of focusing on variations in the symptoms presented by each individual patient. By selecting a remedy that matched the generic symptoms, he was able to successfully treat a large number of patients who had become sick during the epidemic.

Arsenicum album is recommended more as a prophylactic in India. Camphora covers the symptoms of late stages of the illness. There is much debate going on about what exactly is going to be the genus epidemicus for COVID-19.

Arsenicum album 30c is currently recommended by India's ministry of AYUSH, and the homeopaths studying the phenomenon of the COVID-19 pandemic and treating patients have come up with the list of remedies given above that have worked very well to reduce morbidity of their patients. A wide range of remedies that could be used ensures that patients at any stage of infection can be treated successfully. Also, as the symptom picture changes for an infected individual, the remedy can be changed. It is worth noting that in selecting a remedy that matches a set of symptoms or a stage of illness, the homeopath is trying to boost the vital force and not necessarily battle the germs and annihilate them. When the vital force is strong, it does not allow the body to be susceptible to an invading germ.

Dr. Michael Yakir has supported the use of combination remedies if necessary: "Mixtures are only for times of war—or when we have a nation on the verge of death" implying that during the current pandemic that has created an international crisis, we could use a few remedies together in a mixture. Dr. Yakir recommends a kit of a small selection of remedies at home with clear instructions about what to take for prevention, what to take at the onset, and what to take if the situation worsens.[59]

Dr. Sankaran recommends adding one pill of the indicated genus epidemicus remedy, Camphora, to a cup of water and taking a sip every three hours for treatment when the symptoms match.[60]

UNDERSTANDING THE SCOPE AND DEFENDING AGAINST COVID-19 WITH HOMEOPATHY

The COVID-19 pandemic not only created a medical and health emergency—with fever, dry cough, breathing difficulty requiring a ventilator, and pulmonary and cardiac involvement—but in a recent report from China, it is also shown to be causing neurological symptoms in 36.4 percent of very sick patients.[61] The neurological effects involve central as well as peripheral nervous symptoms and can produce dizziness, headache, impaired consciousness, acute cerebrovascular disease, ataxia, and seizure; taste-smell-and-vision impairment, nerve pain, and skeletal-muscular injury. Very sick patients who survive the intensive care, intubation, ventilator, and oxygen mask experience post-ICU trauma (Post Intensive Care syndrome) years after hospitalization.[62] Apart from the initial sets of symptoms and either spontaneous or ICU-based recovery, many patients infected with COVID-19 show a relapse of the symptoms, or they simply do not feel completely well. On retesting, they are sometimes found to have the virus again. It is suspected that the virus goes dormant and reappears when the immune system is at its low point. It is also possible that instead of going dormant, the virus goes away but people get a fresh infection. This implies that they have not developed antibodies to the virus from their earlier infection, or an even more alarming scenario—that newer strains of virus are emerging that are slightly different from the original COVID-19 strain but similar enough to cause the same range of infection in a susceptible and vulnerable host. And because a large number of people are asymptomatic carriers and are testing positive for the virus, they might become reservoirs for the second wave of the pandemic.[63,64,65]

But the physical symptoms of the disease are incomparable to the mass hysteria and a global panic, as per Dr. Jiuan Heng's communication to Dr. Manish Bhatia.[66] People all over the world are collectively experiencing fear of contagion, desire/need for hoarding, mutual suspicion and mistrust, racial backlash, conspiracy, fear of poverty, and fear of loss of work/business/income. Apart from the fear of catching the disease and dying from it, people are afraid for their overall security, well-being, jobs, and even the social structure of their communities. The multiple impacts of the COVID-19 pandemic are yet to be fully reported by psychologists and therapists. How this pandemic will affect the miasmatic aspect of the entire human race is something yet to be discovered by homeopaths.

It is a very heavy price to pay for our unintended exposure to a microbe. As a species, we have been exposed to and we have survived the dark power of many different microbes over our collective history. For some microbes, we have herd immunity (partly due to exposure and partly due to vaccination), but there will likely never be any assurance that humanity will be able to live without the threat of some deadly germ.

Does homeopathy offer any prophylactic support?

For the current COVID-19 pandemic, a few doses of Arsenicum album 30c are recommended by the government of India's Ministry of AYUSH, as a prophylactic. Bhatia[67] has proposed the use of Bryonia alba; and Sankaran has suggested the use of Camphora.[68] For several years Dana Ullman has strongly recommended use of Thymuline for overall enhancement of immunity.[69] At the forefront of homeo-prophy-laxis, Dr. Issac Golden suggests a cocktail preparation of a few remedies and nosodes as a preventive/prophylactic for COVID-19 infection.[70]

The preventive measures put in place by various governments have slowed the spread of the virus, but there is still no assurance that when exposed to the virus, people will not be infected and become symptom-atic. The problem of a re-emergence of the threat has not gone away either. In this situation, homeopathic remedies help reduce the severity and duration of symptoms by strengtheing the Vital Force.

Homeopathic remedies and prophylactic measures are particularly useful because relapse and re-infection in previously infected sick indi-viduals and emergence of slightly different strains of COVID-19 are being reported, and the pharmaceutical/antiviral approach as well as a vaccine are not yet available.

CONCLUSION

As per the report published in the *Lancet*,[71] no vaccines or coronavirus antivirals are available for COVID-19, and therefore non-pharmaceutical interventions are the mainstay in containment of the disease. In this scenario, the alternative, non-pharmaceutical discipline of Homeopathy offers a way out using time-tested remedies that have been successfully used for the past couple of centuries. Current research in Homeopathy even offers a prophylactic solution. If homeopathic support and remedies are available for all those infected with COVID-19, then potentially the asymptomatic carriers and those in early stages of the disease might not progress to the severe stage. As mentioned earlier, the majority of people who get the virus do not become critically ill, so Homeopathy can help them navigate the illness at home and become well without experiencing any nasty side effects, as homeopathic remedies have none. But those with co-morbid conditions, the elderly, the very sick can go to hospitals and ICUs for receiving the latest that the technologically advanced medical science has to offer.[72] Homeopathy can thus take away a huge burden from the hospitals and medical–pharmaceutical industry, particularly because at the moment they have neither the antiviral drugs nor vaccinations available for the public.

If the governments truly want their citizens to receive help with COVID-19 even before the mainstream medicine and vaccine makers can invent and bring their arsenal to the forefront, then governments all over the world will do what India has been doing since 1839: allow Homeopathy to flourish by way of promoting general acceptance, government funding, as well as protection. If truth be told, Homeopathy is way ahead of science.[73] The health and well-being of the public must not be put on hold just because mainstream science is taking its own time (out of fear or ignorance) to catch up with Homeopathy.

In my own observation and study of COVID-19 and how the public has been taught to deal with it, I am reminded of the handwashing and showering rules, as well as the social etiquette of greeting the elderly. These rules were handed down from one generation in my family to the next and were essentially based on the recommendations given in Ayurveda. A daily morning shower and a fresh set of clothes were a must in our childhood home. Another shower before bedtime and a thorough washing of hands, face, and feet several times during the day was a non-negotiable must after we returned from an outing, a social visit, or from school. When greeting the elders, we were not expected to run to them, shake their hands, hug, and kiss them—we were taught to approach them gently, do namaste, bow and touch their feet, stand back at least four feet, and seek their blessings and not talk loudly to their face.

I had often wondered about the reason for these practices and etiquettes. Right now, the much talked-about hygiene practices around COVID-19 have an answer. We collect germs during our sojourn into the world. When we return home, in order not to bring germs, particularly pathogens, into the family, we are taught to maintain a strict routine of washing and showering. Similarly, the elderly folks are known to be a vulnerable population. While moving around in the world, we do pick up microbes, but it is our responsibility to not give these germs to the elderly and make them sick. So, we were taught to not speak to their face (to contain droplets escaping from our mouth), and to stand a few feet away from them so we do not breathe our germs onto their face. By not shaking their hands, we do not pass along the germs from our hands to the elderly. By way of a simple act of maintaining daily routines of personal hygiene and seeking blessings from our elderly, Ayurveda taught us the basic rules for preventing the spread of infectious diseases via droplets. When these rules for maintaining personal hygiene and the social etiquette of greeting the elders were put in place, did the ancients have a deep awareness of the mode of transmission of harmful germs?

It is interesting to note that handwashing to kill germs is an idea that some people have to be taught during the COVID-19 crisis. Though it seems like basic hygiene today, it is a relatively recent discovery in the history of modern medicine. In the early 19th century, even hospitals had no inkling of the importance of cleanliness. They were breeding grounds for infection, often referred to as "houses of death."[74,75,76,77] In this regard, even though Ayurveda is way ahead of the modern times and has long offered clear guidelines for personal and social hygiene, there are a few who ask with a juvenile vehemence for scientific proof for everything from benefits of exposure to sunlight to the importance of exercise.

Medical historian Snowden points out that after World War II "there was real confidence that all infectious diseases were going to be a thing of the past."[78] Chronic and hereditary diseases would remain, but "the infections, the contagions, the pandemics, would no longer exist because of science." Since the 1990s—in particular the avian flu outbreak of 1997—experts have understood that "there are going to be many more epidemic diseases, especially respiratory infections that jump from animals to humans." So, obviously, we might be able to flatten the curve after losing millions of lives and trillions of dollars to the COVID-19 virus, but we are not going to be free from the fear of encountering the next virus that comes up to test our resilience.

What does COVID-19 mean for the global human family?

Harry Van der Jee has proposed that COVID-19 will strengthen the immune system of humanity and thus over the long run improve health and save lives.[79] Human DNA has been built up over millions of years, and in it the genetic information of many bacteria and viruses has been incorporated. Due to all those contributions our physical form has evolved into the amazing instrument it is. Now new information is being offered and the confrontation with this can ultimately only strengthen our collective DNA.

Eventually, when the storm dies down and we are able to breathe normally again without the face masks, we as one species may see that the COVID-19 experience has been globally destructive and at the same time monumentally transformative—just like Shiva, the Lord of creative destruction. Centuries of manmade boundaries between social order, economic muscle, health, religion, philosophy, and ethics (because of resource scarcity the doctors have to decide who gets the ventilator and gets to live and who does not and is left to die!) are stretching, flexing, and extending beyond limits. In some areas, our social structure is crumbling but new forms will emerge. The creative destruction that the management gurus talk about as a part of corporate restructuring is happening right now, not just in one company but on a worldwide scale, to all of us. From this moment of unprecedented transformation, what new form will emerge? What direction will humanity take? Who will be culled from the herd? Who will develop herd immunity and will pass it along to the offspring? As our genetic code is being re-written to accommodate the RNA of COVID-19, how will this newly restructured human genome express itself?

We live in a dynamic and ever-changing scenario. Healing modalities like Ayurveda and Homeopathy are uniquely suited to deal with the extraordinary variables that influence the Vital Force and challenge it to manifest new symptoms and miasmatic expressions.

With its vast arsenal of time-tested and gentle remedies that work on the Vital Force, Homeopathy has a unique approach to the pandemic, as it is able to address not just the symptoms that come up at the physical level but also the emotional symptoms and the extraordinary degree of fear experienced by humanity as a whole. Till the time comes when antivirals and vaccines are invented and COVID-19 is defeated in a military style, people can be helped by Homeopathy and experience a transformation in the expression of their symptoms and the level of their well-being.

Vatsala Sperling, M.S., Ph.D., P.D.Hom., CCH, RSHom (Ph.D. in Clinical Microbiology) served as the chief of clinical microbiology in The CHILDS Trust Hospital, Chennai, India; and as a research scientist, she collaborated with the World Health Organization's International Escherichia and Klebsiella research center. Vatsala Sperling earned her homeopathy degree from The School of Homeopathy, UK, and has been in a successful practice since 2008 (www.Rochesterhomeopathy.com). A published author of ten books (www.InnerTraditions.com) and research papers and articles on homeopathy, spirituality, and healthy living, Vatsala lives with her family in Vermont and spends time in Costa Rica serving on a reforestation project (www.HaciendaRioCote.com).

NOTES

1. John Carter and Venetia Saunders, *Virology: Principles and Applications,* 2nd ed. (Chichester, UK: Wiley, 2013).

2. Samuel Baron, *Medical Microbiology,* 4th ed. (Galveston: University of Texas Medical Branch, 1996).

3. Peter Pollard, "Viruses don't deserve their bad rap: they're the unsung heroes you never see," *Conversation,* October 29, 2015, https://theconversation .com/viruses-dont-deserve-their-bad-rap-theyre-the-unsung-heroes-you -never-see-46887/.

4. Mark Woolhouse et al., "Human viruses: Discovery and emergence," *Philos Trans R Soc Lond B Biol Sci* 367, no. 1604 (October 19, 2012): 2864–71.

5. Nathan D. Wolfe et al., "Origin of major human infectious diseases," *Nature* 447, no. 7142 (May 17, 2007): 279–83.

6. Kasandra Brabaw, "Epidemic vs. Pandemic: What Exactly Is the Difference?" *Health,* March 13, 2020, https://www.health.com/condition/infectious -diseases/epidemic-vs-pandemic.

7. Trisha Torrey, "Difference Between an Epidemic and a Pandemic," *Verywell Health*, May 05, 2020, http://www.verywellhealth.com/difference -between-epidemic-and-pandemic-2615168.

8. Dana Robinson and Ann Battenfield, "The Worst Outbreaks in U.S. History," *Healthline,* March 24, 2020, https://www.healthline.com/health/worst -disease-outbreaks-history/.

9. Vaclav Smil, "A Complete History of Pandemics," *MIT Press Reader,* March 30, 2020, https://thereader.mitpress.mit.edu/a-complete-history -of-pandemics/.

10. Debanjali Bose, "11 ways pandemics have changed the course of human his-

tory, from the over $4 billion spent to fight Ebola to the trillions it might take to tackle the coronavirus," *Business Insider,* March 20, 2020, http:// www.businessinsider.com/pandemics-that-changed-the-course-of-human -history-coronavirus-flu-aids-plague.

11. Anthony R. Fehr and Stanley Perlman, "Coronaviruses: An overview of their replication and pathogenesis," *Coronaviruses* 1282 (February 12, 2015): 1–23, http://www.ncbi.nlm.nih.gov/pmc/articles/PMC4369385.

12. Qun Li et al., "Early Transmission Dynamics in Wuhan, China, of Novel Coronavirus-Infected Pneumonia," *N Engl J Med* 382, no. 13 (January 29, 2020): 1199–207, https://www.nejm.org/doi/full/10.1056/nejmoa2001316.

13. "China Reports First Death From New Coronavirus," *Wall Street Journal*, January 11, 2020, http://www.wsj.com/articles/china-says-person-infected -with-new-coronavirus-has-died-11578709453.

14. Greg Blass, "What can we learn from humanity's long history of pandemics?" *Riverhead LOCAL,* April 5, 2020, http://www.riverheadlocal .com/2020/04/05/what-can-we-learn-from-humanitys-long-history-of -pandemics/.

15. Robinson and Battenfield, "The Worst Outbreaks."

16. Jane Parry, "From SARS to Avian Flu: Vaccines on the Scene," *Scientist,* March 13, 2005, http://www.the-scientist.com/biobusiness/from-sars -to-avian-flu-vaccines-on-the-scene-48986.

17. The History of Vaccines, s.v. "Vaccines for Pandemic Threats," last modified January 10, 2018, https://www.historyofvaccines.org/index.php /content/articles/vaccines-pandemic-threats

18. Yuxian He and Shibo Jiang, "Vaccine design for severe acute respiratory syndrome coronavirus," *Viral Immunol* 18, no. 2 (July 21, 2005): 327–32, https://www.liebertpub.com/doi/10.1089/vim.2005.18.327.

19. World Health Organization, s.v. "Middle East respiratory syndrome corona-virus (MERS-CoV)," http://www.who.int/emergencies/mers-cov/en/.

20. In-Kyu Yoon and Jerome H. Kim, "First clinical trial of a MERS coronavi-rus DNA vaccine," *The Lancet Infectious Diseases* 19, no. 9 (July 24, 2019): 924–25, https://www.thelancet.com/journals/laninf/article/PIIS1473 -3099(19)30397-4/fulltext.

21. Wikipedia, s.v. "Western African Ebola virus epidemic," last modified July 1, 2020, 12:48.

22. Wikipedia, s.v. "2009 swine flu pandemic," last modified June 30, 2020, 08:35.

23. Eun Kim et al., "Microneedle array delivered recombinant coronavirus vaccines: Immunogenicity and rapid translational development," *EBioMedicine* 55, no. 102743 (May 1, 2020), https://www.thelancet.com /pdfs/journals/ebiom/PIIS2352-3964(20)30118-3.pdf

24. Wendong Li et al., "Bats are natural reservoirs for SARS-like coronaviruses," *Science* 310, no. 5748 (October 28, 2005): 676–79.

25. Nsikan Akpan, "New coronavirus can spread between humans—but it started in a wildlife market," *National Geographic,* January 21, 2020, https://www.nationalgeographic.com/science/2020/01/new-coronavirus -spreading-between-humans-how-it-started.

26. Wikipedia, s.v. "Natural reservoir," last modified April 20, 2020, 09:54.

27. Wikipedia, s.v. "2009 swine flu pandemic."

28. Centers for Disease Control and Prevention, s.v. "CDC Seasonal Flu Vaccine Effectiveness Studies," last reviewed July 1, 2020, https://www.cdc .gov/flu/vaccines-work/effectiveness-studies.htm.

29. Lisa Lockerd Maragakis, "Coronavirus Disease 2019 vs. the Flu," website of Johns Hopkins Medicine, last updated July 2, 2020, https://www .hopkinsmedicine.org/health/conditions-and-diseases/coronavirus /coronavirus-disease-2019-vs-the-flu.

30. Stephen A. Lauer et al., "The Incubation Period of Coronavirus Disease 2019 (COVID-19) From Publicly Reported Confirmed Cases: Estimation and Application," *Ann Intern Med* 172, no. 9 (May 5, 2020): 577–82, https://www.annals.org/aim/fullarticle/2762808/incubation -period-coronavirus-disese-2019-covid-19-from-publicly-reported.

31. David L. Heymann and Nahoko Shindo, "Covid-19: What is next for public health?" *Lancet* 395, no. 10224 (February 22, 2020): 542–45, https://www .thelancet.com/journals/lancet/article/PIIS0140-6736(20)30374-3/fulltext.

32. Heymann and Shindo, "Covid-19."

33. Press Information Bureau Delhi, "Advisory for Corona virus," news release no. 1600895, January 29, 2020, https://www.pib.gov.in/PressReleasePage .aspx?PRID=1600895.

34. Julian Winston, "Treatment of Epidemics with Homeopathy—A History," website of the National Center for Homeopathy, https://www.homeopathycenter .org/treatment-epidemics-homeopathy-history.

35. Gustavo Bracho et al., "Large-scale Application of Highly-Diluted Bacteria for Leptospirosis Epidemic Control," *Homeopathy* 99, no. 3 (July 2010): 156–66.

36. Ajoy Kumar Ghosh, "A Short History of the Development of Homeopathy in India," *Homeopathy* 99, no. 2 (April 2010): 130–36, https://www.ncbi.nlm.nih.gov/pubmed/20471616.

37. Abhijit Chakma, "Interesting journey of Homeopathy in India," *Homeobook,* January 30, 2014, https://www.homeobook.com/interesting-journey-of-homeopathy-in-india.

38. Raekha Prasad, "Homeopathy booming in India," *Lancet* 370, no. 9600 (November 17, 2007): 1679–80, https://www.thelancet.com/journals/lancet/article/PIIS0140-6736(07)61709-7/fulltext.

39. Rajendra Prakash Upadhyay and Chaturbhuja Nayak, "Homeopathy emerging as nanomedicine," *Int J High Dilution Res* 10, no. 37 (December 2011): 299–310.

40. Papiya Nandy, "A review of Basic Research on Homeopathy from a physicist's point of view," *Indian J Res Homeopathy* 9, no. 3 (September 30, 2015): 141–51.

41. Prashant Satish Chikramane et al., "Extreme Homeopathic Dilutions Retain Starting Materials: A Nanoparticulate Perspective," *Homeopathy* 99, no. 4 (October 2010): 231–42, https://www.ncbi.nlm.nih.gov/pubmed/20970092.

42. Anisur Rahman Khuda Buksh, "Ultra-highly diluted homeopathic remedies have demonstrable anti-viral effect: A commentary on our published findings related to experimental phage infectivity in bacteria," *Biomed J Sci and Tech Res* 8, no. 5 (September 11, 2018): 6808–12.

43. Ajit Kulkarni, "The Covid-19 Pandemic and Its Homeopathic Approach—Interview with Dr. Ajit Kulkarni," interviewed by Roma Bushimenshy, *Homeopathy for Everyone* 17, no. 3 (March 23, 2020).

44. Douglas M. Borland, *Pneumonias* (Noida, India: B. Jain, 2007).

45. Massimo Mangialavori, "Three remedies I have used for Covid-19," *Homeopathy for Everyone* 17, no. 3 (March 23, 2020).

46. Manish Bhatia, "Coronavirus Covid-19—Analysis of symptoms from confirmed cases with an assessment of possible homeopathic remedies for treatment and prophylaxis," *Dr. Bhatia's Asha Homeopathy* (blog), March 4, 2020, https://www.doctorbhatia.com/treatment/coronavirus-covid-19-symptoms-homeopathic-remedies-for-treatment-and-prophylaxis/?v=7516fd43adaa.

47. Andrew Bogan, "New Data Suggest the Coronavirus Isn't as Deadly as We Thought," *Wall Street Journal,* April 17, 2020, https://www.wsj.com

/articles/new-data-suggest-the-coronavirus-isnt-as-deadly-as-we-thought
-11587155298?mod=searchresults&page=1&pos=1.

48. Julia Ries, "Here's How COVID-19 Compares to Past Outbreaks," *Healthline,* March 12, 2020, https://www.healthline.com/health-news/how -deadly-is-the-coronavirus-compared-to-past-outbreaks.

49. Calvin B. Knerr, *A Repertory of Hering's Guiding Symptoms of Our Materia Medica* (Philadelphia: Davis, 1897).

50. Rajan Sankaran and Aditya Kasariyans, "Homeopathy for Coronavirus Covid-19 Infection," *Homeopathy for Everyone* 17, no. 3 (March 11, 2020), https://www.hpathy.com/homeopathy-papers/homeopathy-for -coronavirus-covid-19-infection/.

51. Rajan Sankaran and Aditya Kasariyans, "Update of the prior study of Homeopathy for Coronavirus Covid-19 Infection in Iran by Dr. Aditya Kasariyans and Dr. Rajan Sankaran," *Homeopathy for Everyone* 17, no. 3 (March 29, 2020), https://www.hpathy.com/homeopathy-papers/update -of-the-prior-study-of-homeopathy-for-coronavirus-covid-19-infection-in -iran-by-dr-aditya-kasariyans-and-dr-rajan-sankaran.

52. Bhawisha Joshi and Sachindra Joshi, personal communication with author, 2020.

53. Dinesh Chauhan, personal communication with author, 2020.

54. Saptarshi Banerjea, "Tackling Covid-19 with Homoeopathy," *Homeopathy for Everyone* 17, no. 3 (March 11, 2020), https://hpathy.com/homeopathy-papers /tackling-covid-19-with-homoeopathy/.

55. Harry van der Zee, "How to boost immunity against coronavirus (COVID 2019)," *Homeopathy for Everyone* 17, no. 3 (March 11, 2020), https://hpathy .com/homeopathy-papers/homeopathy-to-prevent-and-treat-coronavirus -infection-amma-resonance-healing-foundation/.

56. Divya Chabbra, personal communication with author, 2020.

57. Arturo Casadevall and Liise-anne Pirofski, "What Is a Host? Attributes of Individual Susceptibility," *Infection and Immunity* 86, no. 2 (January 2018): 1–12, https://iai.asm.org/content/86/2/e00636-17; Carter, J., Saunders, V. *Virology: Principles and Applications,* 2nd edition, May 2013. http://www .wiley.com/en-us/9781119991427; Baron, S. *Medical Microbiology,* 4th edition, 1997. University of Texas Medical Branch, ASIN: B008UYPLIO.

58. Partha Pratim Pal and Gouri Ningthoujam, "Research Review of Genus Epidemicus," *Int J of Advanced Ayurveda, Yoga, Unani, Siddha and Homeopathy* 8, no. 1 (2019): 545–50.

59. M. Yakir, personal communication, 2020.

60. Rajan Sankaran and Aditya Kasariyans, "Homeopathy for Coronavirus Covid-19 Infection," Homeopathy for Everyone 17, no. 3 (March 11, 2020), https://www.hpathy.com/homeopathy-papers/homeopathy-for-coronavirus -covid-19-infection/; Rajan Sankaran and Aditya Kasariyans, "Update of the prior study of Homeopathy for Coronavirus Covid-19 Infection in Iran by Dr. Aditya Kasariyans and Dr. Rajan Sankaran," Homeopathy for Everyone 17, no. 3 (March 29, 2020), https://www.hpathy.com/homeopathy -papers/update-of-the-prior-study-of-homeopathy-for-coronavirus-covid -19-infection-in -iran-by-dr-aditya-kasariyans-and-dr-rajan-sankaran/.

61. Ling Mao et al., "Neurological Manifestations of Hospitalized Patients With Coronavirus Disease 2019 in Wuhan, China," JAMA Neurology 77, no. 6 (April 10, 2020): 683–90.

62. Annachiara Marra et al., "Co-occurrence of Post-Intensive Care Syndrome Problems Among 406 Survivors of Critical Illness," Crit Care Med 46, no. 9 (September 2018): 1393–401.

63. Dasl Yoon and Timothy W. Martin, "South Korea's New Coronavirus Twist: Recovered Patients Test Positive Again," Wall Street Journal, April 17, 2020, https://www.wsj.com/articles/south-koreas-new-coronavirus-twist -recovered-patients-test-positive-again-11587145248?mod=searchresults &page=1&pos=1.

64. Jeremy Page, "Wuhan Tests Show Coronavirus 'Herd Immunity' Is a Long Way Off," Wall Street Journal, April 16, 2020, https://www.wsj .com/articles/wuhan-starts-testing-to-determine-level-of-immunity-from -coronavirus-11587039175?mod=searchresults&page=1&pos=3.

65. https://www.xinhuanet.com/english/2020-02/13/c_13871178.htm

66. Bhatia, "Remedies for treatment and prophylaxis."

67. Bhatia, "Remedies for treatment and prophylaxis."

68. Sankaran and Kasariyans, "Update of prior study."

69. Dana Ullman, "Homeopathic Medicines for Cough," website of Homeopathic Family Medicine, January 23, 2017, https://homeopathic.com /homeopathic-medicines-for-cough.

70. Isaac Golden, "Preventing COVID19 – How Homeopathy Can Help," Homeopathy for Everyone 17, no. 3 (March 11, 2020), https://hpathy.com /homeopathy-papers/preventing-covid19-how-homeopathy-can-help.

71. Heymann and Shindo, "Covid-19: What Is Next?"

72. Betsy McKay, "Who's Most at Risk From the Coronavirus," Wall Street

Journal, March 14, 2020, https://www.wsj.com/articles/whos-most-at-risk-from-the-coronavirus-11584048476?mod=article_inline.

73. Bill Gray, *Homeopathy: Science or Myth?* Berkeley: North Atlantic Books, 2000.

74. Lindsey Fitzharris, "The Unsung Pioneer of Handwashing," *Wall Street Journal,* March 19, 2020, https://www.wsj.com/articles/the-unsung-pioneer-of-handwashing-11584627614.

75. Katie Camero, "The Do's and Don'ts of Handwashing," *Wall Street Journal,* March 12, 2020, https://www.wsj.com/articles/the-dos-and-donts-of-handwashing-11583952006.

76. Amanda Foreman, "The Long Road to Cleanliness," *Wall Street Journal,* October 4, 2019, https://www.wsj.com/articles/the-long-road-to-cleanliness-11570196433.

77. Grace Paine Terzian, "A Car Key Can Save You From the Virus," *Wall Street Journal,* March 9, 2020, https://www.wsj.com/articles/a-car-key-can-save-you-from-the-virus-11583794581.

78. Jason Willick, "How Epidemics Change Civilizations," *Wall Street Journal,* March 27, 2020, https://www.wsj.com/articles/how-epidemics-change-civilizations-11585350405.

79. van der Zee, "How to boost immunity."

THE INTIMACY OF STRANGERS

Barbara Karlsen

Pushed by the harsh reality of a novel coronavirus, the human species is being forced to realize a new identity. In this new identity everything must be possible—even the intimacy of a "strange visitor" must be possible in it. That is the only courage that is demanded of us, that we trust what is innate within us and love it fearlessly. What is innate within us is a vast organic intelligence that we share with the Earth and other creatures. It is not an intelligence that we imagine from an intellectual point of view, but a far more complex interweaving of different cells, genes, and microbes that shaped the human body. We belong to Nature and we need Nature to actualize the full force of our human becoming. Anything less is to deny the evolutionary forces that shaped us. My point is there is a vast organic intelligence that pervades all of Nature and underlies our development as a species. In thinking we can evolve apart from this intelligence, we have become dangerous to ourselves, and the planet.

When I first met Emilie Conrad in the early '90s the idea that we were an unfolding aspect of the biosphere was so counterculture. However, almost three decades later her vision was never more relevant. It was Emilie Conrad and the practice of Continuum that concretized my initiation into the body as an unfolding aspect of the biosphere. Through the practice of Continuum I came to know the body as a living, breathing process of planetary unfolding—a planetary unfolding that includes the universal memory of all life interwoven into each cell and gene. It was a true initiation into the universal blueprint, a concept that is now a scientific reality thanks to the Human Genome project. We are an immense outpouring of the cosmos. It is not just an intellectual idea; it is molecular, cellular, and visceral scientific reality. It is what lives inside us and actualizes as the immune system that operates as a web of human and ecological relations. It is demanding that we become stewards of the life within us and outside of us. Yes, we may have a human intellect and technical prowess, but we do not possess the wisdom to use it. We have become a serious threat to the whole of our collective existence. Adaptation, evolution, transformation, rebirth, and metamorphosis will be occurring in short order. We need to heed this warning. The message is clear. She will not tolerate us destroying her.

VIRUSES

Viruses are real and cannot be prayed away. We humans have become a climatological and geological force wreaking havoc with all ecosystems and all other species on the planet. Fires didn't stop us, increasing fossil fuel emissions didn't stop us, a pleading Swedish child didn't stop us, melting ice shelves didn't stop us, cancer didn't stop us. It took a virus to stop us. If we don't heed this warning there will be a more virulent strain. We have forgotten that the Earth is our only planetary home. Forget sheltering at home. The Earth *is* our only home. Everyone is being asked to stop, to pause, to reflect. Our survivability as a human species must now include the web of life. This means we can no longer conceptualize genes, organisms, viruses, human beings, or environments separately. We are one body of ecology moving forward.

REORIENTATION

We are in the liminal, the end of one world and beginning of another. How do we begin to orient ourselves to a future that is yet unknown?

How do we begin the work of inhabiting a new self and a new world while sheltering in place? It seems everything prior to this event has suddenly become irrelevant and fallen away. Everything is being re-ordered and re-written. As I strive to make sense of this strange and new world, I yearn for relevant models and symbols to re-orient myself. It seems all of the rational theories fall heavy on my heart. Where does one go to embrace the unfolding wisdom of the liminal? How does one fully plunge into the space of "in between"? As I ask these questions, I am beckoned to dive into the living wisdom of my body. This living wisdom unfolds itself in a direct visceral and cellular knowing that is my birthright. Here movement becomes a space to re-embody the truth of who I am and who I am becoming. My flesh is the Earth and the Earth is my flesh.

INITIATION INTO A UNIVERSAL ONTOLOGY

The coronavirus brings a dose of planet medicine, to ease our ailing Earth. Even our beloved parks, beaches, and trails are closed. We are forced into a world of ritual isolation and solitude. In shamanism illness as well as solitude are symbols of a deep initiation. Sicknesses, dreams, and ecstasies are rites of passage that often constitute an initiation for the tribe, not just the individual. These maladies are meant to cleanse and prepare the initiates for new revelations, as well as for a new world. It is part of the cure.

The initiation we are in right now is begging a new story, as well as a new world. A universal ontology already exists. We just need to live it. Emerging now from modern science is an evolutionary story of interconnection and interdependence with all life forms. We are made of the same stuff as stars, galaxies, soil, microbes, rocks, and redwoods. We are one body of Earth participating in an evolutionary universe. If we ignore this call to our collective awakening, we put at risk the future of our human civilization on our precious planet. The choice is ours.

I am sitting with the numbers of deaths in New York over the last several days, and I am aware that our modern Western culture does not have any initiatory rites and symbols of passage to mark the profound "Initiation" our country is going through right now. As Mircea Eliade wrote in *Rites and Symbols of Initiation: The Mysteries of Birth and Rebirth,* "Initiation is equivalent to a basic change in existential condition; the person emerges from his ordeal endowed with a totally different being from that which he possessed before his initiation; he has become another."

Nothing better expresses the end of an era or the final completion of something than death, just as nothing better expresses the idea of a new life than rebirth. Therefore, the death/rebirth dichotomy serves as a profound archetype and initiation for what we are going through on the planet right now. Before the pandemic, we were turning a blind eye to death but the dying continues. Every 24 hours, 50–200 species of plants, insects, birds, and mammals are becoming extinct. Some call it the sixth mass extinction. This is greater than anything the world has experienced since the vanishing of the dinosaurs nearly 65m years ago. As we enter into this holy weekend of death and resurrection, may we remember the dead and the fallen as the holy initiates. And on this holy occasion, through their initiation and death may the entire world be regenerated and reborn. (Written during Easter 2020)

HOSTING THE VIRUS

If we were to pause and reflect on this crisis as a crucial evolutionary next step, would we host this virus differently? Would we be so quick to eradicate it? Would our immune systems behave differently if we were invited to welcome it instead of fear it? This virus may have a larger role to play in our evolution than we have yet to conceive. That is one of the reasons why I do not feel it was made in a laboratory. Only evolution could have such a profound hand in the total reorganization of our world. How could we humans think up such a plan? Is this the cosmic hand of evolution made visible? And what makes this so radical is that we have no way of knowing what the future holds. The far-reaching implications of the virus are only beginning to unfold, ranging from cosmic (unintended climate benefits), biological (people taking better care of their health), sociocultural (working at home and spending family time together), and financial (economic collapse). It appears we are experiencing a cosmic-size transformation on all levels. Let us make sure this cosmic transformation is not brushed over too quickly in an attempt to return to a normal that was far from normal.

VIRUS AS A CATALYST

I don't think the coronavirus is here to "kill us." I believe the coronavirus is here as a catalyst to awaken positive change on this planet as we move forward. The most urgent crisis facing humanity today is not the coronavirus but the destruction of our only planetary home and its ongoing effect on our human health. Looking at the statistics we see that all kinds of illnesses are increasing, not just epidemics but also cancer, heart disease, and other chronic diseases. Something is really wrong. We live in a momentous time. The significance of changing the way we steward the planet has never been more crucial. Medical systems will not be equipped to handle the surge of diseases that we will see unfold in our lifetime if we do not change our behavior on a global scale. We are being called to a new order and understanding of life. This new life requires that we awaken to a new reality of how everything in the universe is interconnected and interdependent. We can no longer operate from a lesser order. This means recognizing that although we feel special, even unique as human beings, our DNA is only one gene pool among many more in the biosphere.

ECO-PSYCHIC AILMENTS

Individually and collectively we are experiencing feelings of fear, anger, overwhelm, and grief on a scale that we have never seen before. With so many individuals and families experiencing the loss of health and livelihood, our hearts are broken on a daily basis and stretched beyond their capacity to feel. We don't know where to turn. We feel powerless. Many are calling this the age of ecological collapse, and it will come with a whole new set of psychological problems that we have never seen before. When the place we call home is burned down or flooded, or when we lose our health to an invisible threat, the mix of fear, grief, and increasing uncertainty takes an emotional toll on our body-mind and soul. We need to grieve and confront our painful feelings. This creates the space for something new to emerge. And the new requires a total reorganization of everything that preceded it.

OCCUPATION OF THE BODY IN THE COVID-19 CRISIS; A WAR ON BODILY AUTHORITY AND AGENCY

In my Continuum class this morning on Zoom, participants courageously expressed a bodily felt sense of the imposed restrictions of a prolonged shelter-in-place. This imposed restriction is not so much about the virus as it is about the control of our bodily nature and agency. Yes, there are dangers involving true threats, I know that. But there are also dangers to the expression of a primordial wisdom and agency that is our birthright. How do we know who we are when our world falls apart? Who are we becoming? These questions are not answered by reason alone. These are answers that reveal themselves in the deepest crevices of our human species wisdom—a human species wisdom that expresses itself in the reorganization of everything that came before. Call it adaptation, evolution, or rebirth. It doesn't matter. The body will know before the mind what the next species will be.

IMMUNITY

I see the current crisis of COVID-19 as an outdated understanding of the human body, immunity, and its connection to the web of life. And because we can see interdependency in a way that we couldn't see it before (thanks to shelter-in-place and masks), I believe the capacity for real change now exists. There has been a lack of tending to the body of the Earth and to the wild nature of our human bodies. This has affected our immunity and our soul. Immunity is not something that develops in isolation from the human soul behind a mask, or in a sanitized existence. Immunity arises in a life well lived and emerges in the commitment to live the largest human story we are capable of living. I believe the time has arrived to up-level our human story and destiny. We are living too small.

GERM THEORY VERSUS TERRAIN THEORY

This pandemic is getting more and more disorienting as times goes on. It wasn't bad enough that we had to shelter in place, isolate from each other, and conduct our lives through technological objects. But now we are being told to wear our masks even when outside. On a gorgeous spring day yesterday, I saw people of all ages biking in masks and walking in Nature with masks. Are we willing to accept this definition of life? Isn't that why we evolved for hundreds of thousands of years alongside the EARTH? The paradox of the situation is that our bodies are dealing with viruses all the time. That is part of the crucial role they play in the development and evolution of our immune system. Our human genome is outsourcing Nature all the time, including viruses, for important genetic information. One has to wonder if the current pandemic is here to illuminate a much larger pandemic: the lost interdependence between humans and Nature.

SUMMARY OF MAIN POINTS

Our extreme self-centeredness and degradation of the planet have brought untold ecological carnage, the greatest threat of which is to our bodily selves. With the overuse of antibiotics, vaccines, and the mass spraying of synthetic pesticides, we have wreaked havoc not only with the planet but with our own body ecology. Everyone is in a desperate rush to boost their immune system against an invisible invader. This illusion of a separate human from Nature is dangerous and in the end will destroy us if we continue to act Godlike, manipulating DNA, and spraying pesticides so that we can better control ourselves and other living beings.

Far from being superior to microbes on the evolutionary ladder, it now appears that microbes and bacteria are not only the building blocks of life but occupy more space and mass than us humans. And the bottom line is, they mutate and evolve more rapidly . . . hence the novel coronavirus jumping from animal to human. This realization shows that they are ready to mutate and alter themselves and the rest of life should we humans be so foolish as to annihilate the planet and ourselves. Maybe it is time we collaborate with our microbial ancestors instead of killing them, for clues to our own survival.

UNITY WITH THE COSMOS

We may know less about this pandemic than we think we know. And we may be approaching it in entirely the wrong way because we think we know. We are using an old paradigm called germ theory and categorizing COVID into outdated models (reductionist), hence the mortality rates. Maybe it is not just another coronavirus at all. Maybe this novel virus is the "genetic bits" of a cosmos striving to bring forth a supreme birth, one that the human intellect alone could not have given.

Just like the sea creatures found themselves thrust up on the burning shores of a new land, Nature may be attempting to evolve a new species in us and through us. However it occurred, let this be our quantum leap to the beginning of a new planetary era. This is a different path for perfecting the human, and it has nothing to do with intellectual theories, psychology, or imposing a technological existence upon the human body. It is about forging a magical unity with the cosmos.

BARBARA KARLSEN is a Continuum movement teacher, nurse, and somatic psychotherapist trained in birth psychology. She graduated from Naropa University in Boulder with a master's degree in somatic psychology, and she did her doctorate at the California Institute of Integral Studies. Her areas of special interest and study have been in Earth-based spirituality and ancient Buddhist psychology. She has a private practice in Marin County, California, where she teaches and practices the shamanic art of Continuum and re-birthing. Other supportive services include working with core body issues such as attachment, intimacy, and sexuality through somatic awareness, resourcing, and support. For more information go to barbarakarlsen.com.

CORONA YOGA

Staying Sane in Crazy Times

Joel and Michelle Levey

The word *yoga* means to unite or join together as in a "yoke." Could the global pandemic of the coronavirus actually be a "crown of union" shining light on the reality that "All related we are . . . All family we are . . . All together we are . . ."? We are indeed being called to come back into union, to connect deeply within ourselves—the path of true healing—and re-member our deep interconnectedness with each other, with Nature, and with all living beings. Like yoga, this journey we are all on together can be a path of transformation, a path of healing and wholeness, and a way of becoming stronger, more resilient, more tolerant. And like all spiritual paths, the way begins inside each of us.

> *One world is dying,*
> *and another is being born.*
> *Let's tend to both of them with compassion.*
> —Marianne Williamson[1]

We are immersed in an ocean of global uncertainty, flooded by feelings of vulnerability and overwhelm, confined to "sheltering in place," subject to physical distancing, social isolation, and social rebellion, while at the same time many of our familiar escape routes from the usual irritations and frustrations of daily life have been cut off or reduced. As a result, many of us have not been able to avoid coming face to face with the persistent and sometimes terrifying presence of our "inner enemies" parading through the narrow corridors of our minds and acting out in defiance in cities around the globe.

We are clearly in a time of crisis and disruption. The global CV-19 ordeal has provided countless dangers and opportunities—as the Chinese character for "crisis" implies. While this may be one of the most significant global crises we have seen in our lifetimes it will likely not be the last. The lessons we learn now and the strengths we develop will serve as our wisest investments for the future.

As many of us are seeing for ourselves in such potent and dangerous times, our minds can become our greatest ally or most dreaded enemy. In times of crisis our skill in managing our minds, or lack thereof, can either liberate and guide us in ways that are beneficial to ourselves and others, or debilitate and destroy us and those we are with.

When we (the authors) were invited to develop the once-secret Jedi Warrior Training Program for the U.S. Special Forces, our charter was to teach teams of the most technically sophisticated and well-equipped warriors to "recognize and befriend their inner enemies and stop the war inside." One of the primary axioms of this intensive six-month full-time immersion training program was "You can only manage what you monitor." Jedi Warrior grew out of our work with the U.S. Army's legendary "First Earth Battalion" task-force, which envisioned how a new generation of soldiers equipped with extra-ordinary skills and the ethics of warrior monks would become an Earth-stewarding force-for-good. While this inspiring vision was greatly influential, its potential has yet to be fully realized within the military. These notes are meant in part to enlist *you* in this noble endeavor!

While in decades past, disciplines of personal mastery such as martial arts, meditation, and mindfulness may have been primarily for elite teams or the privileged few, in times of crisis like these, traditions of deep transformational learning are essential for everyone seeking to maintain their health, sanity, and care for others in order to survive and flourish.

When confronted with the tremendous challenges of leading her people in direct actions to stop the powerful tar sands oil pipeline interests from coming into and polluting the Salish Sea near Vancouver, Amy George, daughter of the great Chief Dan George of the Tsleil-Waututh Nation in British Columbia, inspired her people by saying, "It's time for us to warrior up!"

Our colleague, Otto Scharmer, a Senior Lecturer at the MIT Sloan School of Management, offers this insight, "We live in a profound moment of disruption. And disruption comes with pain and grief, and also comes with a gift. And the gift is that the moment that disruption hits we can have a glimpse of awareness of what it truly is that is essential for us."

The following pages offer a guide to essential skills to help you find the courage, capacity, and commitment necessary to "warrior up," to grow stronger, wiser, and more resilient in the midst of challenge, and to even thrive as we step into a world that continues to change in often bewildering ways. May you take these offerings to heart and find inspiration and strength in weaving these ideas and skillful means into the fabric of your life.

The insights and teachings in this chapter are inspired by our combined 100 years of intensive research and study of the inner sciences and technologies from many modern and ancient wisdom traditions, and informed by our experience as clinicians running pain clinics and stress mastery clinics in large medical centers, as well as our work with leaders, teams, organizations, universities, and communities in many nations around the world. The data make it clear that disciplining the mind is profoundly effective for everyone, particularly those serving in the military and frontline services (medical, fire, police, rescue, etc.) and dedicated caregivers. We all need techniques to liberate ourselves from being dominated by anxiety, depression, grief, vulnerability, and burnout.

We were recently invited to give a special briefing on our Jedi Warrior Program at a special conference at British Parliament on The Vital Role of Mindfulness for the Military and Emergency Blue Light Services. As we listened to the other colleagues and presenters speaking of their experiences living and working in war zones, in ambulance, police, and fire services, it was clear that most of these brave and committed professionals had endured tremendous trauma and had suffered greatly. It was inspiring to hear them speak of how learning to practice mindfulness had helped them find skillful ways to embrace and liberate themselves from being dominated by anxiety, depression, burnout, grief, and vulnerability. Through their own experiences in resurrecting themselves from their own suffering, they had then been inspired and motivated to make this type of training and deep education available for their colleagues and soldiers in arms.

Most people have had very little experience or study in understanding the true nature and potential of their mind and therefore have never really learned to manage their mind very well. To do this we must understand and discover what the mind actually is.

DISCOVERING THE MIND'S TRUE NATURE

The human mind has two primary dimensions and functions. The surface or relative dimension of the mind is related to the activity and contents of the mind, and functions to represent our world through a myriad of different forms in a creative display of thoughts, mental images, perceptions, and feelings. These comprise the energy and information of the mind. Each of the many types or "species" of mental activity is a momentary, impermanent, evanescent experience.

The second dimension of the mind, known as the "nature of mind," is a deeper, more universal or ultimate dimension that has been described by many terms in both modern and ancient traditions and is related to our capacity for "awareness" and "knowing." Because this inner knowing has no color, shape, or form, this deeper dimension of mind is so subtle, elusive, and ungraspable that very few people fully realize the profound significance of this essential dimension of their being in their lifetime. The nature of mind is boundless and clear like the sky, within which the cavalcade of fleeting, impermanent experiences of the relative mind come and go like "clouds" or "winds" arising, dissolving, and passing through the vastness of space. This dimension of the nature of mind is like a domain of consciousness that abides within a quantum realm of reality prior to the manifestation of measurable waveforms that appear in the relative Newtonian universe. It is this dimension of mind that allows us to monitor and manage the contents and creative activity of the relative mind.

Once you develop the capacity to experientially embrace both these dimensions of mind in a unified, integrated manner, your access to the deeper nature of mind opens portals of possibility. Simply put, with awareness you have choice. With awareness you discover that anxiety is an option . . . reactivity is an option . . . and, kindness is an option. . . . With awareness you can channel your creative mind powers away from dominating obsessive patterns of thought into more creative and productive mind-states that empower and ennoble rather than deplete and debilitate.

BEFRIEND AND MANAGE YOUR MIND

During times of crisis, isolation, or absence of distraction, many people default to allowing their minds to spin out of control, perhaps lapsing into incessant worry. Depending on how skillfully we monitor and manage the creative nature of our minds, we can either drive ourselves crazy or move into states of profound well-being and pro-social engagement. David Chethlahe Paladin, a Navajo friend and teacher of ours, often reminded us that "Worryin' is just prayin' backwards." Our creative imagination, if properly utilized, can be a powerful force to find strength, hope, clear direction, and meaning in difficult situations.

In a recent response to the Covid-19 crisis, the Dalai Lama wrote, "I take great solace in the following wise advice to examine the problems before us: If there is something to be done—do it, without any need to worry; if there's nothing to be done, worrying about it further will not help."[2]

One of the best strategies we have found for managing worry is to practice worrying intentionally! How do you do this? Simply set a time each day to devote yourself to worrying. At the appointed time, sit down and call forth any specific worries that come to mind, and give these concerns your undivided attention for 10 to 15 minutes. If during this time any pleasant or positive thoughts come to mind, simply let them go and turn your attention back to your worries. And then, when your time is up, just say to your worries, "I'm terribly sorry, but our time for today is over, and I have many other meaningful things to attend to now. If you are still relevant and need my attention again, I'll check in with you tomorrow at the same time. Have a nice day." *Poof!* Then, as you get on with your life, if any worries intrude into your mind-space at other times during the day, simply say to them, "I see you—and you are early for our appointment." Alternatively, you can simply click and drag that worry into an "I'll think about this later" file on your mental desktop, and carry on with your life!

For many people this simple mind-management strategy has been a game changer, liberating them from being dominated by intrusive worrisome thoughts.

ONE BY ONE . . .

Another example of a skillful way to harness and direct the creative power of our minds is inspired by a dear, wise, elder friend. An avid explorer of the nature of mind for many decades, Gladys discovered that one of her best strategies for managing the creative activity of her mind during wakeful times in the middle of the night was to pray for her nearly two-dozen grandchildren, one by one. She noted that this gave her peace of mind and ease in her body, and that she seldom made it through her whole list of grandkids before she drifted back into a peaceful sleep. Consider how you might adapt this strategy in your own life (even if you don't have twenty-four grandchildren!).

MANAGING THE STORIES WE TELL OURSELVES

Because our bodies respond equally to mental images as to sensory ones, learning to monitor and manage our thoughts is an essential life skill, especially during times of crisis.

A powerful mind-management technique comes from a tribe in Africa that we learned about from our colleague Angeles Arrien, a cultural anthropologist. Angie relayed that from an early age, children in the villages are trained to be mindful of their thinking. If they became aware of a foreboding thought like, "Oh no, what if there is a lion hiding behind that tree waiting to eat me?" they learned first to recognize and then release the thought by saying to themselves, "And this is a story that doesn't need to happen!"

In this day and age this may translate into recognizing thoughts like "I'm going to get sick and die," or "I'll never find a new job," or "my investments will be worthless," as "stories that don't need to happen."

This practice is balanced by appreciating that we also have positive stories that come to mind, and that when we are mindful of positive thoughts we can make a mental note of "Ah, and this is a healing story." The children in this African tribe were also trained to recognize and note helpful and reassuring thoughts in this way. Now, for example, when you are mindful of thoughts like "my child or friend is going to recover from this illness," or "the seeds I planted in my garden will grow strong and feed my family this summer," or "my friends will be there for me when I need them," you can smile to yourself and say, ". . . and this is a healing story."

This mind-management technique is a treasure and so easy to use.

ALWAYS BEGIN WITH GRATITUDE

In times of great emotional or social upheaval, the practice of gratitude is especially essential and effective in helping us, both individually and collectively, to bring ourselves into harmony and balance. Opening our hearts and minds to gratitude helps to dissolve the illusion of our sense of isolation or insufficiency by remembering and affirming how profoundly held, supported, and nourished we are by people around us and by the universe at large.

If you run out of reasons to feel grateful, remember the wisdom of the Zen teacher Thich Nhat Hahn, who reminds us that we can even be grateful for our "non-toothache" (all thirty-two of them!) as well as for all the other calamities that are not currently present in our lives, families, or community.

In the wisdom ways of Indigenous people, and in the annals of medical science, the balancing and restorative power of gratitude is deeply revered. Giving thanks is traditionally the first step for many Indigenous communities whenever they gather for meetings or ceremonies. Across the ages and across the globe, the intentional cultivation of an attitude of gratitude holds a central place in the daily practices of a wide variety of people and contemplative traditions.

Many of our teachers remind us that gratitude is an essential practice for living in balance. Some say that when we generate gratitude in our hearts and minds we complete the circle between ourselves and the source we are grateful for. With this sacred hoop of gratitude in place, it ensures that those circumstances causing us to feel grateful will continue to flow in our lives. On the other hand, if we don't generate gratitude for the gifts of our lives, we break this circle and the causes of gratitude will cease to flow. In these ways, gratitude opens our hearts and minds to a deeper sense of connection, the deep, meaningful, and nourishing relationships and dynamic balance that allow us to thrive.

Gratitude infuses us with the strength to open our hearts more deeply in order to touch the vulnerability and suffering that may arise when what we love, value, cherish, or care about inevitably changes, decays, or fades away from our lives. This recognition opens our hearts to compassion. In this way, our beloved friend and teacher Joanna Macy suggests that if we are seeking to understand and wisely respond to the complex and challenging circumstances in our lives, world, families, or communities that we should always "begin with gratitude." Beginning with gratitude gives us access to the strengths and resources that we need to embrace the challenging aspects of our lives and world, to see them with our wisdom eyes, and to go forth with greater wisdom, compassion, and effectiveness. Gratitude anchors us in goodness and the precious, though fleeting, gifts of our lives. In doing so, we release our tensions and calm our anxieties and fear. For a brief yet precious moment we can relax and rest in a greater sense of wholeness, harmony, balance, and relatedness.

Gratefulness can be a way of life, a meditation, an attitude, or a practice. Since gratitude is such a direct path to experiencing a more balanced state, we'd like to offer a simple yet powerful practice. In designing and teaching the Mindfulness and Meditation Laboratory program for Google, we found that this meditation was the number-one favorite of the Googlers, because it is direct, simple, can take as much or as little time as you wish to give it, and delivers immediate positive and stress-reducing results.

We teach this practice as a way to remember the many gifts, blessings, resources, and allies of our lives worthy of our attention in the spirit of gratitude and thanksgiving. It has also been shared by circles of friends, families, and communities around the world at times of Thanksgiving, and we invite you to share this practice with your loved ones and friends as well.

Here's how the practice goes:

As you begin, reach up, touch your heart, and gently smile to yourself with a tender sense of deep connection and deep reflection. Allow the flow of your mindful clear presence to blend with the natural rhythms of your breath, and allow yourself to simply settle into this state of open awareness and rhythmic, flowing sensations.

As you become more fully present now, bring your attention to your heart as you call to mind anyone and anything in your life that you are grateful for. As you inhale, gather whoever or whatever comes to mind into focus in your heart, reflecting upon your gratitude for them. Breathing out, let your heartfelt gratitude flow to them and through them as waves of blessings. Let your mindfulness savor and embrace the imagery, feelings, emotions, and sensations associated with this experience of gratitude for this person or this aspect of your life. Be mindful of how this presents itself to you. Rest in this contemplation as long as you like, and when you feel complete, release your focus on this aspect of gratitude and welcome whoever or whatever else next comes to mind that you are grateful for. . . . Gather them into your heart and radiate your gratitude, thanksgiving, and blessing back to them.

Let each unique experience of gratitude and blessings be taken to heart, one by one, like counting beads on a mala or rosary. Continue in this contemplation as long as you like, gathering anyone or anything that you are grateful for, radiating your gratitude and blessings to them, one at a time or all together.

You can rest in this contemplation for as long as you like or have time for, allowing each breath to bring to mind a loved one, a friend, or someone who has been kind to you, someone who is teaching you patience or how to forgive. . . . Allow each breath to shine from the depths of your being through the depths of their being in order to light up their life with your gratitude, love, and compassion.

Taking these many gifts to heart, complete and affirm the circle with gratitude, ensuring that the stream of blessings and deep connections in your life and in the universe will be unbroken. This sense of deep connection and deep relatedness is the primary ground in which balance is rooted.

As we open our hearts to gratitude, we are better able to listen and sense more deeply into the tender dimensions of our hearts. Opening our wisdom eyes to see, sense, and commune with the deeper, subtler dimensions of our lives, we discern that even within gratitude, there may be overtones of sadness, disappointment, regret, vulnerability, or grief that are all inseparable from our gratitude. Gratitude helps us to embrace the many dimensions of our lives more deeply and gives us the insight and strength to open our hearts more fully to compassion for ourselves, and for others.

HONORING OUR TEARS

You know that you're close to the truth when you have tears in your eyes.

—GOPI KRISHNA,
MYSTIC, SOCIAL REFORMER, ENGINEER

Be mindful of moments when your eyes moisten and honor these moments. Remember that tears flow when we are close to the Truth. Normalize your tears and take these precious moments to heart with gratitude, celebrating these encounters with your humanity! As Joanna Macy reminds us, "Our sorrow is the other face of love, for we only mourn what we deeply care for. . . . The sorrow, grief, and rage you feel is a measure of your humanity and your evolutionary maturity. As your heart breaks open there will be room for the world to heal."

CLEAR MIND DON'T KNOW

Having the courage to welcome and embrace uncertainty is a profound strength. While most people spend their lives trying to avoid uncertainty, times of disruption and crisis provide a fierce opportunity to embrace and befriend uncertainty. We learned a powerful practice to accomplish this from one of our Korean Zen teachers, Soen Sa Nim. Here's how it works:

Breathing in, silently say to yourself "Clear mind, clear mind, clear mind . . ."

Breathing out, say, "Don't know")))))))

Continue on, breath by breath, phrase by phrase, for some time. . . .

Clear mind, clear mind, clear mind. . . . Don't know)))

Note: In our style of writing))) represents an expansion, extension, a ripple effect.

Allow this practice to help you access and gain confidence, strength, clarity, and courage from your inner clear mind . . . and to discover the profound human resources of surrender, humility, and creative potential that arise when you embrace uncertainty.

ZOOM FATIGUE

Now that our normal means of connecting in the social sphere and outer world have been curtailed, we are more immersed than ever in social media and the web. Sheltering in place, people are flocking to the internet and stacking their schedules with online Zoom meetings, classes, webinars, family meet-ups, yoga classes, ad infinitum. As a result, many people are suffering from Zoom, web, or screen fatigue. In many ways this intensified reliance on the web is drawing us away from ourselves without offering the true nourishment of heartfelt human contact and warmth of meaningful social connectivity, or connection with ourselves.

As people of all ages are "skilling up" to retool and adapt to this new communication reality, here are some novel inner-tech moves and online disciplines to help avoid web burnout and Zoom fatigue:

- Before each online session, pause, take three mindful breaths, listen for your intention, and clarify—what is driving you to get back online? Are you bored and looking for stimulation or distraction? Is there a question, hope, or fear that is leading you to search for information? Are you seeking connection—and if so—

what motivation is driving you to seek that connection?

- If you have a tendency to tumble aimlessly around the web, clicking here and there, set the intention to be mindful of clicking links—i.e., to notice the physical movement and sensation of touching and moving your cursor and clicking. This will help ground you in present-moment awareness and embodied experience.

- Before you send a message or email, or finalize a post, pause to reflect for a moment on the impact you would like it to have in the hearts and minds of the people who open it; and as you click or press "send" or "post" with your finger, transmit the spark of this intention along with your message.

- Whenever you read a bit of news, pause for a moment before you go on to the next bit to be mindful of what feelings, thoughts, and desires have been activated within you through encountering this information. Give it a moment to sink in and digest.

- If you read about individuals, or groups of people who are suffering or who have died, pause for a few moments to let your heart reach out to them like you are shining a lighthouse beam of loving kindness, compassion, or comfort to them from your heart. Trust that this care is conveyed and received. Do this with the same kind of confidence and certainty of effect and impact as you would have in sending a digital message to an individual or group. In fact, there are thousands of excellent research studies that confirm the reality of these "non-local effects."

- When you are finished surfing the web, pause for a few moments to quietly return to resting in the mindfulness of the natural flow of your breathing and notice what thoughts, mental images, and emotional feelings are most present and alive within you. Reflect on this web session and be mindful of what was worthwhile, enriching, or worthy of remembering, and what really wasn't worthy of the precious time, energy, and life force that you invested. Take these lessons to heart and carry them forward with you.

CONNECTING WITH MORE OF OURSELVES

A principle found in various traditions of ecosystem management and self-management is that if a living system is compromised, suffering, or diseased, the remedy will be found by connecting it with more of itself. As we expand our hearts and minds to connect more deeply with the world and the beings around us, our health and vitality will be increased. We can certainly do this even when we are physically isolated, so here are some perspectives and methods to help you to accomplish this.

RECEIVING AND RADIATING

A human being is part of the whole called by us 'universe', a part limited in time and space. We experience ourselves, our thoughts and feelings, as something separate from the rest. A kind of optical delusion of consciousness. This delusion is a kind of prison for us, restricting us to our personal desires and to affection for a few persons nearest to us. Our task must be to free ourselves from this prison by widening our circle of compassion to embrace all living creatures and the whole of nature in all of its beauty.

—Albert Einstein

Just as the relatively small and limited area of an island has a massive yet invisible foundation connected to the whole of the earth, each of us has access to an inconceivable wealth of resources that flow to us and through us from the boundless wholeness that connects us with all things and all beings. Though we may have lived with a delusional self-image that is impoverished in its scope, with curiosity and practice we can widen the circles of our wisdom and compassion to embrace an ever broader sense of our wholeness and deep relatedness to all life. On the next page is a practice that we have found helpful for cultivating this.

Resting in the easy natural flow of your breathing, reach up, touch your heart, and smile with a tender sense of deep connection and deep reflection. Give thanks for the blessings and opportunities of your life and dedicate yourself to living ever more deeply in the compassionate spirit of balance that you sense is most essential to your true being. Allow your mindful awareness to blend more deeply now with the natural rhythms of your breathing and settle into this state of deep connection and flow.

As you sit here now, envision yourself sitting at this center of your universe, surrounded by all living beings. Holding this image in mind, pause for a moment to remember, invite, or sense the presence of those who have most deeply inspired you with their examples of compassion in action. These may be people you know, teachers, mentors, or family members, or people you have read about in scripture, books, or discovered on the web.

Reach out from your heart, and with your hands, to these beings whose inspiring presence in your life is truly a blessing, a source of renewal, deep information, and strength. Imagine that all of them are right here with you now, surrounding you and shining like a constellation of radiant compassionate suns. Or if you like, envision that these many sources of compassion merge into a single brighter star that shines a radiance of compassion and blessings into your life.

Imagine that with each breath you reach out to them, and they reach back to you. Envision yourself holding their hands; and through your connection with them, sense that you can draw strength and inspiration to deepen your sense of wisdom, compassion, and balance. Notice how the stronger and more sincere your own aspiration, the deeper and stronger the flow of inspiration streaming to you and through you becomes. With each breath receive this light and inspiration, and radiate your gratitude back to each of them. Receiving . . . and radiating . . . with each breath.

Imagine now that each of these inspiring people in turn reaches out to hold the hands of those to whom they look for guidance, strength, and compassion, and that they in turn reach out to those who have inspired them. Sense your teachers reaching out to their teachers who reach out to their teachers, who reach out to their teachers. . . . Your ancestors, reaching out to their ancestors, reaching out to their ancestors. . . . Envision yourself balanced within and receiving from this endless cascade of wisdom, compassion, and inspiration as it flows to you and through you from countless inspired ancestors of the far and distant past.

Sense this inspiration flowing to you as the light of wisdom, blessings, or compassion, soaking into you, illuminating and empowering you. It energizes the parts of you where your life force is weak. It balances whatever needs to be balanced and heals whatever needs healing. This light floods, cleanses, and opens the spaces and places within you that are clogged or congested, and nourishes the seeds of your deepest potentials to blossom in your learning how to live in balance. Like sunlight filtering into a deep clear pool, sense these waves of inspiring grace flooding your body-mind-energy-spirit. Every dimension of your being is illuminated, blessed, balanced, and renewed.

With each in-breath you are filled, saying silently to yourself *"receiving."* Envision that with each exhalation you can *radiate* and expand this circle of gratitude, extending balancing and harmonizing energies with each out-breath. Receiving with each inhalation . . . and radiating with each exhalation. . . .

Breathing in, imagine the inspiration and blessings flowing into you, filling your heart, infusing your whole body and being. Breathing out, sense, imagine, or feel that your heart is silently radiating balancing and harmonizing qualities of being like a bright, shining star. Effortlessly offer the natural radiance to inspire all beings to live in greater harmony and balance. Allow it to shine out through the darkness within or around you. Allow the light of your influence to effortlessly illumine your inner and outer world. Let this be the light of your presence, the light of balance, the light of peace, the light of goodwill and compassion.

Now, as you sit here at this center of your universe, surrounded by all living beings, envision yourself reaching out to those who look to you as a source of inspiration, guidance, or loving support and imagine each of them reaching back to you. Reach out to your children, to your friends, to your family, to your students, clients or customers, to your patients, and to all those who look to you as they seek greater balance, belonging, or well-being in their lives. Receiving compassion, inspiration, wisdom, and strength from those you draw guidance from, reach out with your hands and from your heart, and allow each exhalation to radiate harmony and balance to those who, in turn, look to you. Let each inhalation bring you inspiration from the sources of strength you are aligning and attuning to, and allow each inhalation to also gather the gratitude that streams back to you from those that look to you as a source of strength and inspiration. Receiving . . . and radiating . . . with each breath.

Envision each person you reach out to receiving the harmonizing and balancing influence you offer to them and taking the light of your love, strength, or compassion to heart. Sense that this deeply touches, strengthens, and inspires each of them. As your compassion reaches out to your children, envision them receiving and taking this light to heart and then passing it on to their children, who pass it on to their children, who pass it on to their children and to all whose lives they touch directly or indirectly. Envision your students reaching out to their students who reach out to their students. Imagine that all those to whom you reach out take this light of your qualities of being and compassion to heart, and pass it on to those who will pass it on in an endless cascade of inspiration and blessings that reaches out into the world to help affirm and presence the light of compassion for countless generations to come.

In this way, receiving and radiating, sense yourself balanced in the infinite expanse of "deep time," surrounded by all beings, reaching out from this fleeting moment where all the experiences of the infinite past and all the potential for the boundless future converge. Viewed in this light, realize that your real life-work is to truly balance yourself in order to increase your capacity to reach out and realize your connectedness and wholeness, to increase your capacity to gather inspiration, wisdom and compassion, to take it to heart, and to then expand this circle of light, strength, love, and compassion to all beings. With each breath, receiving and radiating, expand your circle of harmony, balance, peace, compassion, and well-being for the benefit of all beings.

MINDFULNESS, COURAGE, EMPATHY, AND COMPASSION

The word EMPATHY is derived from the ancient Greek empatheia, which was formed from the words for in and pathos. A century ago, German philosophers borrowed empatheia to create the German word Einfühlung, "feeling into," which was later translated into the English word empathy. Interpersonal empathy describes the capacity that nearly all of us have to include another being into our awareness in a way that enables us to sense what they might be experiencing physically, emotionally, and cognitively. Empathy, literally taken, is feeling into another, while compassion is feeling for another, accompanied by the aspiration to take action that benefits the other. Empathy is often a precursor to compassion and part of compassion, but it is not compassion. Whereas empathy is a good thing in the right dose, I believe that we cannot overdose on compassion.

—Joan Halifax[3]

As human beings we are biologically designed to be deeply resonant with and attuned to other living beings and the world around us. Learning to read the subtle cues and signals from our environment, from other human beings and other creatures, has been the key to our survival and development for millions of years. While our ability to be empathically attuned or resonant with others is a precious gift that ensures our success in forming deep bonds and meaningful relationships with others, if we become empathically overwhelmed by the suffering, pain, trauma, and vulnerability that we encounter, we are in danger of experiencing burnout, or what many people in the past have described as "compassion fatigue."

A wealth of recent research demonstrates that the so-called "compassion fatigue" is actually a misnomer and does not really exist. This condition is more accurately described as "empathy fatigue" or "empathic distress." The shift from empathy to compassion can be understood by observing the pathways and regions of the brain that are activated when we are empathically attuned to the needs and sufferings of others. These regions of our brain are adjacent to and deeply entangled with the areas of our brain that light up when we ourselves are suffering or in pain. When we shift from empathic resonance to compassionate responsiveness, the empathically attuned regions of our brain quiet down, and a completely different set of neural circuits is activated as compassion comes online. This movement to compassion relieves our empathic distress and activates a visceral sense of well-being, relatedness, peace of mind, aliveness, and prosocial fulfillment.

The good news is that the remedy and protection from empathic distress or overwhelm is readily accessible by shifting into compassion. The emerging research illuminates three essential elements of compassion:

1. Noticing the suffering of others (Mindfulness);
2. Empathically resonating with the suffering or pain of others as a feeling within ourselves (Empathic Resonance); and
3. Engaging in action to ease the suffering and reduce the causes of suffering (Compassionate Responsiveness).

Archbishop Desmond Tutu reflected this wisdom when he said, "Compassion is not just feeling with someone, but seeking to change the situation. Frequently people think compassion and love are merely sentimental. No! They are very demanding. If you are going to be compassionate, be prepared for action!"

When compassion is engaged and embodied in action, it may be expressed by reaching out from our hearts with kindness . . . offering food, shelter, protection to others in need . . . speaking kind and helpful words . . . or reaching out from our hearts with loving kindness, blessing, or healing thoughts or prayers. These are all examples of being moved into responsive compassionate engagement that can protect us from the dangers of being empathically overwhelmed by the suffering in our lives and world. Given the likelihood that waves of challenging disruptions will continue to escalate throughout the duration of our lives and for generations to come, the current wave of disruption reminds us that we would be wise to develop our capacity to embrace and respond to the challenges and opportunities that our emerging new life and world will bring.

TONGLEN, THE BREATH OF COMPASSION

Compassion is a natural response to the suffering in our lives and world. It is an active response that emerges when we are balanced in the face of suffering and moved to alleviate that suffering. For our compassion to be effective and not create more problems it must be guided by wisdom; and for wisdom to deepen, courage is required—the courage to keep looking ever more deeply into the web of complex, subtle, and meaningful interrelationships that weave the fabric of our lives and world.

The transformative practice that follows is one of the most powerful methods for opening our hearts and minds to compassion—for ourselves and for other beings. This practice, woven on the loom of the breath, fuels this fire of compassion with wisdom, love, and dedication. We call it "the breath of compassion." This meditation, called *tonglen* in Tibetan, comes from the Buddhist tradition, though it can also be understood as the natural impulse of a mother who, moved by compassion for the fear or suffering of her child, wishes to take in and transform her child's suffering and give back her love, strength, and healing energy. The word *tonglen* literally means "taking and sending." The practice of *tonglen* teaches us to embody this same natural gesture in working with our own pain and suffering, that of our loved ones, and all suffering beings. It is widely regarded as the ultimate practice for opening our hearts fully to compassion and for dissolving fear and separation. In our work we teach this practice widely, especially for people who work as caregivers or who offer protective services to others.

The Essence of the Practice

As you breathe in now, envision that you can gather the raw energy of any agitation or discomfort you may find in your body or mind, drawing it into the transformational vortex of your heart center like fuel for a furnace—and then, out of compassion, let that suffering fuel the fire of transformation, giving you more light of compassion to radiate. With each breath, breathe in compost and breathe out flowers and fruit. Breathe in fear, and let its energy be released into the radiance of confidence on the exhalation. Breathe in imbalance, and let it too fuel the radiance of your steadiness and resilience. Radiate the light of compassion out on the waves of your breath as a blessing of balance and peace in the lives of all those who share your world.

In this way, with practice, you will begin to understand that as you learn to embrace the difficult, challenging, or painful experiences of your life and work, this actually gives you strength and becomes a vehicle to find the courage, wisdom, and power to open your heart ever more widely and deeply to compassion. When you are faced with fear and suffering, let it fuel the radiance of your compassion for yourself and for others who "just like me" suffer in similar ways. Faced with beauty and the sweetness of life, let it intensify the radiance of your gratitude and joy. Imagine yourself as a light-bearer of wisdom, strength, and compassion illuminating and protecting the goodness of the world. Imagine the silent light of your innermost being blazing with radiant compassion in countless helpful ways. Holding your loved ones and friends in mind, radiate this light to them. Bring to heart and mind the leaders of the world, the children of the world, the beleaguered nations and species of the world, and radiate your heartfelt compassion and care to them.

Of all the contemplations that we know of, this "breath of compassion" practice is without equal in its universally practical applications and profound implications for learning to live ever more deeply in the flow of dynamic balance. Taken to heart, this practice, which rests in the natural rhythms of your breath, refines the balance of our sense of inner and outer, self and others, me and we, joy and sadness, pleasure and pain, peace and turbulence. The power of this practice helps us expand and affirm our intimate interrelationship with all of life, awakens our generative compassionate capabilities, and activates a genuine heartfelt concern for the well-being of others who, just like you, want to be happy and free from suffering.

More Detail on This Meditation of Tonglen

As you begin, brighten the light of your clear presence with a gentle, heartfelt smile, and touch your heart to activate and affirm your connection with the light of compassion that shines from the depths of your being. Then allow this clear presence and great compassion to move with the natural rhythm, flow, and balance of your breathing.

Resting in the natural flow of your breathing, allow the area of your chest around your heart center to relax, open, and soften, and establish a clear sense of inner spaciousness, like a vast open sky. Imagine or feel yourself as completely open and clear inside, like a big body balloon. Totally open and pervaded with the clear light of mindful awareness, you have a deep sense of being completely transparent inside, that the space within you is continuous with the space around you. It is as though all the pores of your body are totally permeable to the flow of air and currents of energy that pass in and out through you, and you feel almost as if you can breathe in and out of all your pores. Pause and rest here until you can clearly establish this feeling of open, clear, and unobstructed inner spaciousness.

Then sense that within the region of your physical heart is a dimension of your true, pure, noble heart—your heart center or chakra. Sense or imagine this as a stainless dimension of deep inner strength, purity, and compassionate presence. Classically this dimension is symbolized as the sacred heart, or the pure heart jewel, whose light shines forth with limitless loving kindness and compassion embracing all beings. In this contemplation you can also envision this dimension of the heart as a transformational vortex, where you can draw in the fire of suffering and turn it into the pure light of radiant compassion and well-being.

One of our teachers, Geshe Gyaltsen, often called this practice "Hoover vacuum cleaner meditation!" Powered by the motivation of compassion, use the "motor" of your inhalation to work like a "Hoover" suction, gathering up and drawing into the transformational vortex of this pure dimension of the heart any pain or negativity that might be present in your physical, mental, emotional, or spiritual continuum. If you don't feel any particular discomfort at the present moment, simply let your inhalation draw in any seeds or latencies that may be lying dormant in your body or mind—potentials of future suffering that could ripen if conditions became right. You can envision these as heavy, hot energy, or dark smoke.

Breathing in heat or the fire of suffering and pain, let it dissolve into this pure dimension of your true heart, and sense that the suffering is completely dissolved and resolved, and then ride the waves of the out-breath to radiate cooling waves of compassion, comfort, and ease back to where the suffering came from.

As you exhale, imagine that from your heart center waves of clear, radiant, healing light pour forth. Imagine these waves filling your whole body and mind, healing, energizing, and transforming you. Allow the vortex at your heart to function as an energy transformer drawing in negativity, darkness, or pain and transforming it into radiant light and healing energy. For example, drawing in agitation as you inhale, let it dissolve into the pure dimension of the heart, and radiate peace back as you exhale; drawing in anger on the in-breath, let it dissolve, and radiate patience and compassion mounted on the waves of the out-breath. If you've taken the suffering of *fear in* with your breath, now send back *faith* and *strength* with your *out*-breath. If the pain you breathed in was *tension*, let it dissolve, and breathe back *relaxation*, and so on. "Breathing in hot and heavy . . . breathing out cool and light. . . ."

Some people find it helpful to visualize a color, texture, image, or sound that carries the feeling of the quality they are sending. Others prefer to simply ripple out a pure clear wave of intention. The key is to allow each breath to deepen and affirm your sense of being capable of this compassionate transformation in the pure dimension of the heart.

Continue in this way, embracing, gathering, sweeping and vacuuming, resolving and transforming, mounted on the waves of the breath, for as long as you like. Remember to keep your breathing gentle and natural, not forcing or holding the breath in any way. As you practice, you may find that the grosser, more noticeable discomforts dissolve or change. As this happens, allow your awareness to be drawn to subtler and subtler messages that call for your compassionate attention.

The *tonglen* meditation is a contemplative analogue of the Saint Francis prayer, which is rich in similar imagery and intent:

> *"Lord, make me an instrument of thy peace.*
> *Where there is hatred, let me sow love;*
> *Where there is injury, pardon;*
> *Where there is doubt, faith;*
> *Where there is despair, hope;*
> *Where there is darkness, light;*
> *Where there is sadness, joy.*
> *O Divine Master, grant that I may not so much seek*
> *to be consoled as to console,*
> *To be understood as to understand,*
> *To be loved as to love.*
> *For it's in giving that we receive, and it's in pardoning*

> *that we are pardoned.*
> *And it's in dying—that we are born into eternal life."*
> —SAINT FRANCIS

The true power of this meditation comes alive as you begin to realize that the radius of your compassion can be vast and limitless in its scope, and that you are able to receive and transform the energies of others who share the larger body of life with you. The larger the field of connection and interrelationship that you acknowledge and participate in, the greater will be the reservoir of resource you have to draw from.

As you deepen in this practice, you realize that just as you wish to be free of the pain in your back, your loneliness, or heartache, so too does the person in the seat or house, the office, village, or country next to you, or across the world. And you also realize that it really doesn't take any extra effort at all as you breathe in to hold the compassionate intention to embrace and transform their suffering at the same time as you're breathing in and transforming your own.

If you are tormented by anger or grief, imagine and affirm that with each breath, as your compassion transforms these energies or feelings within the sphere of your own personal, local body or mind, those same feelings shared by others can be embraced and transformed by your compassion as well. Envision and affirm that the radiance of this compassion emanates out through you to be received by anyone who shares the same feelings, who suffers in the same way, or who even has the latency for such vulnerability or disease in the future. (Note: In an age of current or future pandemics, meditating in this way to reduce the latency for disease can be very powerful.) Whatever the form of distress or suffering you find within yourself, embrace that in others or in the world at large.

When it feels natural, allow the circle of your compassion to expand to embrace anyone else who comes to mind: a friend or loved one, a neighbor or coworker, a whole group of vulnerable people, or other beings who are living with fear, suffering, disease, or danger. Breathing in, allow your heart to open, to touch, receive, embrace, and transform the fear, the distress, the loneliness, grief, or suffering. Allow these sorrows or distresses to dissolve and resolve completely within the pure, open, limitless dimension of your true heart. As this transformation naturally unfolds, allow the energy of your heartfelt compassion to also dissolve or explode the optical delusion of a separate self, and expand your sense of identity and balance in the larger field of being that includes all life. As you feel the sensations of your out-breath, allow your heart to naturally open to send back waves of peace, patience, calm, protection, loving kindness, and radiant compassion to all who suffer. Experience the openness and connectedness that awaken as you expand the circle of your active, engaged compassion, caring, and balance in this way.

Continue to deepen into this meditation for as long as you like or have time for, allowing each cycle of breaths to further deepen and affirm your capacity to open your heart and expand the circle of your compassion.

This contemplation can be done in many different situations. First start with yourself, then let the circle of your compassionate awareness reach out to others yearning for the same quality of peace, harmony, and well-being that you're looking for, and keep expanding the circle of your compassion to individuals, groups, or other living beings who come to mind.

Taken to heart, this practice of *tonglen* can become a profoundly integrative practice for living in balance as you move through the world. In the Mahayana tradition it is said that once one begins to sense that their true life, identity, and purpose are intimately related to all living beings, and one begins to cultivate this mode of higher-order relationship and balance in relation to all beings, one's capacity to engage in this meditation naturally and intuitively expands until in the moment of completely awakening to one's true nature and highest potentials, all that is left is a selfless quality of presence that exists in the mode of *tonglen* for the benefit of all beings.

Once you understand how this practice works, you can weave it into the flow of your daily life. Quietly and invisibly while you are sitting alone in your home, watching or reading the news, walking down the street, shopping, waiting for or riding on public transportation, driving in your car, being present during a particularly tense conversation—know that this meditative mode of being is available to you. This way of being is well suited for living in dynamic balance with a spirit of compassionate engagement in your world. It offers a glimpse of how it might be to become a beacon of inspiring, balancing, and healing presence as you move through the world.

We've taught this practice to tens of thousands of people from all walks of life, and of different philosophical and spiritual inclinations: to medical staff working in clinics and emergency rooms, to Special Forces troops facing untold dangers and fear, to children, corporate executives, clergy, and world-class athletes. For some, this practice makes immediate intuitive sense from what they know of the unobstructed flow of energy and information in the natural world. Others will translate this practice into a deeply personal participation in God's love or the compassionate presence of Quan Yin radiating and extending from the pure, sacred dimension of their heart out into the world.

As we traveled and taught in Asia, we found that this practice of *tonglen* is especially accessible for our Asian students who grew up with a sense of connection to Quan Yin, "She Who Hears the Cries of the World," as the embodiment of universal compassion. For those of us with the faith, intuition, or experience to know that there is a dimension of pure-heartedness within us that is stainless and virtually invulnerable to any sort of discordant energies, the sense of offering the cries of the suffering world to the heart of your own inner Quan Yin can be as natural as breathing in and receiving, and breathing out and radiating compassion to all beings. One beloved Christian colleague who had practiced *tonglen* for many years wrote a profound sermon for his congregation musing how likely it was that the final contemplation of Jesus on the Cross might have been in the spirit of *tonglen,* taking in and transforming the ignorance and sins of all beings who had "missed the mark" (the original meaning of the Hebrew word for "sin") and dedicating all his love and compassion to their salvation—be they in the historical time of Jesus, or in future times when his teachings were still present in our world.

The spirit of this practice of "taking and sending" is as universal as the wish of a mother to take upon herself the suffering of her child and to offer all her strength, love, and joy to comfort them. Each of us will translate this potentiality in our own way. In this spirit, we invite you to take this sage advice to heart, practice it in your unique way, and see how it speaks to and lives through you.

Keep in mind that whether you are visibly able to transform the sufferings of others through this practice is secondary to transforming the illusion of your own sense of separateness and the task of dissolving your own fear and narrow self-protectiveness. The real power of this meditation practice lies in developing a deeper experience of kinship with the beings of the world, and in breaking free from our preoccupation with our own personal situation or limited personal identity.

Tonglen is essentially a mind training that empowers our inner access to qualities of balance, and an immense source of compassionate transformational potential. It can awaken the wisdom and compassion necessary to free us from the anxiety, fear, imbalance, and exhaustion that come from trying to vainly protect the illusion of a separate self. It teaches us to live in harmony and balance within a more expansive, generative, and universal view of wholeness, and to honor and deeply respect the sacred mystery of interdependence by seeing how activating compassionate regard for others works simultaneously to heal our relationship with ourselves as well.

INTEGRATION: RECEIVING AND RADIATING
COMBINED WITH *TONGLEN*

With practice, you may come to naturally realize that with each breath, you can gather the light, strength, power, blessings of all creation, add your light to that, and then radiate and offer it to all beings.

With each breath we can align and attune ourselves with all the sources of guidance and blessings available in our lives and world, back through endless time, and we then can radiate, offer, and extend those streams of blessings and inspiration to those who look to us, and through them to all who look to them, and through them to all who look to them.

With each breath we can gather into the pure depths of our true heart the pain of all the fires of ignorance, greed, and aggression raging in our world, and we can transform, dissolve, and resolve those raging fires in the deep, clear pool of our heart, and radiate the cool, clear, radiance of compassion, balance, and harmony into the hearts and souls of others.

Freed from the ignorance and fear that breeds in the shadows of the optical delusion of consciousness that leads us to sense or view ourselves as separate from the world and all beings, we are ennobled and empowered to open our hearts and mind, our wisdom eyes and pure hearts, to become sacred vessels of transformation capable of embracing and transforming our relationship to the sufferings of the world.

And, in those inevitable moments where the darkness or complexity of our lives or world overwhelms us, we can also reach out to hold the hands, or draw into us the hearts of all the ennobling beings we receive and draw light and inspiration from, and we can blend those streams of empowering light with the torrents of grief, pain, or sorrow that we are tapping into.

Understood and taken to heart in this way, we realize that with each breath, 21,600 times a day we can balance ourselves, stand strong, shine bright, dispel fear, and connect with streams of sustaining and life-affirming strength, blessings, and inspiration, and that we can extend our light, love, and strength out to others. In this way we balance and weave together with each breath the practices of receiving, transforming, and radiating.

HOLDING LOVED ONES IN OUR HEARTS

The secret of my song though near,
none can see, and none can hear.
And, oh for a friend to know the sign
And mingle all their soul with mine.

—RUMI

Some years ago, we had the good fortune to participate in an intensive year-long silent contemplative retreat. As a couple, we lived in separate rooms and had very little contact with each other or with any of the other participants in the retreat. Other than an occasional deep bow, or rare hug on the path to the dining room, we had no physical contact, and we had only a few hours' worth of actual conversation during the entire year. Yet, each day at five o'clock in the afternoon, we had a "date" and would shift our attention from the contemplations that were the focus of our retreat, to hold each other in heart and mind. Merging together like two spheres of light, we would rest in the light of each other's love as if we were two beings sharing one heart and looking out through each other's eyes. It was often a deeply moving and affirming connection that left each of us uplifted and amazed; and honestly, looking back at the depth of connection we felt with each other, it was strangely the most intimate year of our lives together.

In this disruptive time of physical distancing and isolation, when we are likely to be separated from loved ones and friends for long periods of time, this heart-to-heart meditation can be extremely meaningful and profoundly healing. You can either do this practice on your own, merging your heart and mind with a loved one or friend, or you can set a date with a loved one to "meet up" and do this practice together at a specific time each day.

As a couple, when we are physically apart for any length of time, we have continued to set a time each day to sit together and hold each other in our hearts. During this time, we reach out to each other from our hearts and let ourselves merge to share a common heart and core. In a state of deep, intimate connectedness, we rest in the radiance of the love we share. We allow the light of our love for each other to radiate out to others as an offering and a prayer that will strengthen them in whatever they need at that time.

Even though we may be away from each other for some time, when we come back together, we usually feel closer than ever before. When we are home or traveling together, we often make some time to sit quietly together in this way and carry this sense of deep connectedness into our busy day and work in the world. Many people we work with have taken this example to heart and have developed a similar practice that they share with their partners, parents, children, grandchildren, or beloved friends. The results are always inspiring.

GUIDELINES FOR STAYING SANE IN DISRUPTIVE TIMES

Establishing a suite of daily practices can provide a sense of stability, grounding, harmony, balance, and flow to our lives—especially in times of disruption. Though this requires minimal time it can deliver tremendous value to your life. These disciplines will give you a stronger foundation to stand upon in the face of change, challenge, and uncertainty by supporting and encouraging you to be more mindful throughout the day, be clear on your priorities, and make wiser choices.

Begin Your Day in a M.A.G.I.C.A.L. Way

We have created this unique sequence of contemplations as a wonderful way to start each day. Begin with the very first moment of the day that you are "awake" to being awake– ideally *before* you get involved in any way with your devices. This becomes a liberating way of declaring your sovereignty over your devices by giving priority attention to your primary operating system—the deep nature of your own mind-body-spirit. Here are the contemplations:

M indful of your Embodiment . . . breathe in . . . and out . . . a few times to feel and affirm your physical aliveness.

A wake awareness! Tune in to this quality of "awake awareness"—the deep ground of your being.

G ratitude. Be mindful of whomever or whatever you are grateful for, taking them to heart, with gratitude overflowing as blessings for these precious gifts in your life.

I ntention. Listen for guidance to clarify your personal intention for the day; be mindful how this guidance comes to you—as words, images, feeling, knowing. . . . Add to this personal intention a "Universal harmonic" of that intention in the sense of "for the benefit of all"—i.e., may I be peaceful so that all beings who share the larger body of life with me have access to greater peace . . . may I be courageous today, so that all beings may have access to greater courage. . . . Remember this intention throughout the day to help you to "live on purpose."

C onnection. Draw strength from remembering that you live within a seamless wholeness and constellation of all the forces and sources of inspiration that support you. For a few moments simply breathe, receiving and radiating waves of inspiration, strength, gratitude, and blessings with each breath, affirming these meaningful connections.

A wareness. With an "ahhh" relax and rest in clear, boundless, sky-like awake-awareness. Affirm this most essential dimension and ground of your being.

L ove. Sensing deeper into boundless awareness, discover that it is inseparable from boundless love extending to and embracing all beings . . . and let it shine.

Having aligned and attuned to these qualities, carry this on into your day in a "magical" way!

NOTE: This practice can telescope in time, meaning that once you are familiar with how it works, you can do it very quickly or take a longer time to really savor each element more deeply.

Throughout the Day

Be mindful of where your attention goes.

Whenever you notice that you have lapsed into mindlessness and distraction, smile to yourself . . . reach up and touch your heart . . . and "re-boot" your mindful-clear-presence by simply softly sighing (((Ahhhhh)))

Then . . . remember and re-affirm your intention for the day.

With that guidance clearly in mind, proceed to live "on purpose" and bring your mindful, clear presence to whatever you are doing and to whomever you are with.

Repeat this again and again throughout the day.

Evening Reflections

Toward the end of each day, make some time to reflect on your day using the "Four Rivers." The Four Rivers practice is inspired by the wisdom of the Basque people, who say that if you "swim in these rivers every day" you will live a fulfilled and meaningful life with greater vitality.

Pause to reflect. . . . Where today were you. . . .
- Challenged?
- Surprised?
- Inspired?
- Deeply Moved or Touched?

You can journal with these questions, and also share these with friends or family over a meal, or in a shared social media group each day to inspire and support each other.

SHARING KINDNESS

These times of radical disruption in our lives have the potential to bring out the best in us and the worst in us. Knowing that we have access to skills and frames of reference necessary to embrace the waves of change and challenge and to find opportunities in these changes is a profound gift. Appreciating the strengths and vulnerabilities of ourselves can help us to recognize and honor the strengths and vulnerabilities of others. The simplest and most direct way to put this wisdom into practice is kindness. This excerpt from Naomi Shihab Nye's brilliant poem "Kindness" seems a perfect way to conclude this chapter.

Before you know what kindness really is
you must lose things,
feel the future dissolve in a moment
like salt in a weakened broth.

What you held in your hand,
what you counted and carefully saved,
all this must go so you know
how desolate the landscape can be
between the regions of kindness . . .

. . . Before you know kindness as the deepest thing inside,
You must know sorrow
as the other deepest thing.
You must wake up with sorrow.
You must speak to it till your voice
catches the thread of all sorrows
and you see the size of the cloth.
Then it is only kindness that makes sense anymore,
only kindness that ties your shoes
and sends you out into the day
to mail letters and purchase bread,

only kindness that raises its head
from the crowd of the world to say
it is I you have been looking for,
and then goes with you every where
like a shadow or a friend.

JOEL LEVEY, PH.D., and MICHELLE LEVEY, M.A., cofounders of Wisdom at Work, are globally recognized pioneers introducing resilience, mindfulness, and contemplative sciences into a wide spectrum of mainstream organizations. They have served as directors of clinical stress management programs for large medical centers and faculty for University of Minnesota Medical School. Over the past 40 years their work has inspired diverse audiences in hundreds of leading organizations around the globe including: NASA, Google, World Government Summit, British Parliament, and M.D. Anderson Cancer Research Center. Based in Seattle and Hawaii, Michelle and Joel's published works include: *Living in Balance: A Mindful Guide for Thriving in a Complex World; Mindfulness, Meditation, and Mind-Fitness;* and *Wisdom at Work.* Learn more at:

http://WisdomAtWork.com/MindfulnessPioneers/

NOTES

1. Marianne Williamson (@marwilliamson), "One world is dying," Twitter, October 12, 2011.
2. Dalai Lama, "A Special Message from His Holiness the Dalai Lama," the website of His Holiness the 14th Dalai Lama of Tibet, March 30, 2020, https://www.dalailama.com/news/2020/a-special-message-from -his-holiness-the-dalai-lama/amp
3. Joan Halifax, *Standing at the Edge: Finding Freedom Where Fear and Courage Meet* (New York: Flatiron Books, 2018), https://us.macmillan.com /books/9781250101341.

ATTAINING OUR BIRTHRIGHT

Steve Curtin

Always said that if I had the time I would start writing.
Well, with the quarantine, I am suddenly blessed with an
abundance of that rare commodity called time.

The Human Being is a wondrously designed sensory mechanism. Our bodies are constantly working to keep our internal physiology in a state of balance as we interact with the world around us. We are in a continual state of communication with an incredible amount of information in each moment. The external environment is constantly shifting as we move through it, bringing us into relationship with an ever-changing sea of information, yet the internal state remains basically constant or in a dynamic equilibrium with our environment. Body temperature, blood pH, heart rate, breath rate, interchange of body fluids all have to stay within a very tight range regardless of the stresses our environment subjects us to. Just think of some of the outside forces we must adapt to—changing temperatures, barometric pressure, relative humidity, and noise or light levels are a few that come to mind. Rarely do we have any awareness of all this work going on right inside our own skin. The only time we might pay any attention is when something goes wrong.

In addition to dealing with external environmental changes, the body also has to respond to whatever is taken into the system. Many of the things presented to the internal environment are life supporting or designed to help our bodies (i.e., food, water, or air). Every time we take in food or drink this presents the system with more work. It must break down these objects so they can be digested, absorbed, and then transported to the appropriate location to bring nutrition and build up the tissues. Afterward the waste products of metabolism must be excreted in the form of feces or urine.

Earth's atmosphere is made up of a myriad of gases. It is composed of 78 percent nitrogen, 20 percent oxygen, 0.9 percent argon, 0.04 percent carbon dioxide, about 1 percent water vapor, and a minute amount of other gases. With every breath in, the lung amazingly has a mechanism to selectively absorb oxygen and expire carbon dioxide. Oxygen then is transported via red blood cells to be used in cellular energy (ATP) formation. Once again, the whole system has to maintain physiologic homeostasis. An incredible array of actions takes place, mediated by our autonomic nervous system, to keep blood sugar, body pH, temperature, and body hydration in a constant state. Not one ounce of energy needs to be spent on conscious thought to accomplish all of these actions. Every time I reflect on the workings of our bodies I am humbled. My thought is, what an amazing design of creation!

It is my intention in my writings to explore the ways of aiding ourselves, and all of Life on this wonderful planet, to maintain our Innate Health. I believe that as one begins to be more aware of the intelligence inherent in life, that individual will be able to interact in a more conscious way to help create Balance and Harmony in our environment, rather than the discord we are seeing today. It is my prayer and fervent hope that the Human species can step back into our birthright, which is to be servants of that Intelligence in creating a Home that supports all of life to attain Its highest potential.

A FORGOTTEN RELATIONSHIP

As I sat comfortably at the base of the willow tree, the sun was warming my back, which was resting against the trunk. I had just completed leading a session in a workshop entitled "Awakening the Wild," intended to help the participants open their sensory perception to experience the world around them in a deeper way. At this moment I was participating in the next exercise directed by one of the other workshop leaders. This session was using music and body movement to come into a deeper sensing of our bodies. All the participants had headphones on with a music set designed to quiet one's mind and thereby facilitate the sensate experience. I had walked slowly, moving in sync with the sounds coming through the headphones, along a wooded dirt path in the bird sanctuary in which our retreat was being held. Rather abruptly, an inner voice directed me to sit, to rest against a fifty-foot-high, beautiful, mature willow tree. A gentle sea breeze was blowing in off the nearby beach, causing the tree to sway. This motion against my spine created a very subtle massaging of my vertebral column, deepening my state of comfort and ease. Music soothing my ears, along with the subtle ministrations that the tree was performing on my back, helped to lessen the usual noises in my body and mind, which serve to continually distract me from the communication with what is present in each moment.

I felt a tugging on my awareness, directing my attention to the grass on which I was sitting. I could feel all the activity of life contained in the grass around me. There was so much alive in that square yard of grass around my body, where just a minute ago I noticed nothing. I felt myself drawn into the roots of the grass. I sensed an intelligence totally different from my own, awakening in me a remembrance of a time long past . . . a time when we had an intimate deep connection. It felt like a portal opened at that moment, and I and the grass merged into one consciousness. This perception extended through all the interconnected roots for miles around. As I synchronized with this field of awareness, I felt a collective gasp! It was not coming from me. The grass was shocked that a human being was communicating with it. The realization of this stunned me.

Initially the grass was frightened by the intrusion of this human interaction, but slowly we actually began to converse. It shared a memory from a distant past where all humans were interconnected with it—not with words, mind you. The communication was on a primal, deep sensate level, the way all of life on this planet has interacted for eons. It is a form of communication that humans partook in long ago before our present enculturation dulled our senses.

Once the grass recovered from its initial shock, they welcomed me back, as one would welcome back a relative who has been gone on a very long trip. Life on this planet, actually the planet itself, has patiently waited for our return. I was welcomed back into a world of interconnected life— a web of all living beings in a state of constant interaction and cohabitation. We are all parts of a huge living being, and we all have important interrelated functions to keep this incredible Earth vibrant and healthy. I traveled through the roots of the grasses to meet many other members of the vegetal world who coexist in this magnificent world. No words were exchanged, but I could feel an outpouring of information flowing toward me, as if it were being downloaded directly into my being to be digested later. As I slowly came back into awareness of my body sitting at the base of the tree, I came to realize that only twenty minutes had passed. I felt like I had been there for days. I pledged to reread the story of Rip Van Winkle, as I understood in a different way that mystifying story of a man who supposedly slept for years at the base of a tree.

STEVE CURTIN began his osteopathic general practice in Brunswick, Maine, in 1992. He currently practices in the Sanctuary on Church Street in Ellsworth, Maine, a space that he founded for the merger of osteopathy, yoga, Ayurveda, chi gung. Of it, he writes, "It has long been my intention in my work to aid in the process of awakening each individual the initial 'Breath of Health.' This center is an expression of that desire to be of service to HEALTH manifesting more fully in all of us. It is my prayer that the creation of this space helps all who enter its boundaries."

DECONSTRUCTIONS, DIVINATIONS, AND VISIONS

TITANIC NATION, COVID WAKE

Eric Myers

The wounded Ship of State adrift, no novel status, a 3,000-mile-long gash ripped into its starboard side as the vessel pushes past the iceberg and lists through choppy cultural waters churning with invisible viral predators—every soul now a sailor into the Great Unknown.

(COVID-19 is not the iceberg. But it does riddle the waves.)

The communal limbs of the conscripted crew ripped akimbo, social dismemberment of the New Normal assimilated on all decks, whether for Lord or Lower Class, previously unthinkable acts of psycho-social auto-amputation now become a daily ritual—out of fear that charting this course, turbulent though it may be, is far better than subsumption by infested waters.

(COVID-19 is not the triage surgeon. But it oversees the operation.)

Online illumination our only portholes to the world and to each other, a postmodern perversion of the prophecy of digital deliverance, forced entry into mediated reality rather than the open invitation to the liberating virtuality it promised in the long-lost Way-Back-When—before plague-ridden hooves galloped out from the Good Book and revelated themselves into our reality.

(COVID-19 is not the medium. But it is, perhaps, the message.)

Having hit the iceberg some time ago, long before the "invisible enemy" of COVID-19 arrived to exploit the sundering, the Bardo Ship of American State lurches on, everyone onboard for the isolation as the vessel begins its descent. The passengers ignore the sinking feeling that accompanies the physical dip, distracting themselves instead with the hope that their social and economic selves can be sutured back together one day down in the sick bay, stitched into a Frankensteinian patchwork man that at least suggests the previous corpus socialis. But, like any amputee, everyone knows it won't be the same after this—at least not for a long while—whether they can consciously acknowledge that knowing or not. Because some things are not to be gotten over—they can only be gotten used to.

A lost limb.

A lost love.

A lost life.

Or a faith lost in a previously impervious ship, formerly guided by providence but now slowly sinking down down down, the heart of its hull crucified by a mountainous spear of ice, innards exposed to an invisible army amassing all around.

And as the boat bobs on the waves, COVID-19 speaks. It is assuredly no gift, but it might be a mage, visiting us from afar and offering sidereal inspiration, so that we may plot a different course through the darkness of the deep.

I have referred to the United States as "Titanic Nation" since the mid-1990s; collectively, we had hit the self-summoned iceberg of our own eventual demise. And it was only a matter of time before the slow-motion sinking would be complete, with or without the type of novel threat COVID presents. Perhaps a generation. Perhaps a century. Maybe even more.

Regardless of the timeline, it seemed clear there was no way for a culture so adrift to thrive, let alone survive, at least not without a radical transformation of its current incarnation and its underlying cultural coding—a transformation that seemed unlikely, barring intervention on a providential scale or a hail Mary, all-humans-on-deck rallying cry. The ship is still beautiful, if ragged. The ship is still beloved, if beleaguered. The ship is not beyond repair, while the animal kingdom's boon of timelessness does not apply to any rescue plan.

Despite all of that, none of this text constitutes a demeaning of ostensible American ideals or a blithe dismissal of what the nation is "all about." Patriotism is not constrained to cheerleading, and the most vocal criticism often comes from a fervent love of what America espouses itself to be—and a deep sadness at the reverse alchemy wrought upon the cruise of the country, and thus the world. Gold turned to garbage, the theoretical perfection of a Declaration transduced down into the perversion of its practice.

Titanic Nation would not be taken out by an icy aggregation of extrinsic forces. It would not, most likely, be invaded or assimilated by a foreign culture, since the Cold War was won and hegemonic empire entrenched. It could not even be pillaged by a pandemic, as long as its immune system was intact. This was not the nature of its disaster. Instead, it was an inside job. The culture's reason had slept and it would devour its own kind like Goya's Saturn—or devour itself, an Ouroboran entity choking on its tail without the promise of regeneration from the ingestion. Our own Hungry Ghost, believed to be banished by our national supremacy but in fact externalized and disavowed and cast into the shadow through our not-knowing, would gobble us up in an act of ectoplasmic auto-cannibalism that would leave behind nothing but a skeleton of our former vitality. The nation had conjured its own iceberg and inflicted its own injuries, non-dualistically acting as both perpetrator and victim, subject to the destructive manifestations of traits that before, in a purer form, had culminated in historic triumphalism. The reasons for this self-sinking, the layers of the cultural iceberg so to speak, were as numerous as they weren't numinous. Let's interrogate only three, in no particular order, since it's never easy to see what hulks below and what rises above:

1) THE ICE OF ISOLATION

The almost religious belief in unbridled American freedom and individualism, to the exclusion or at least diminution of the collective welfare: the go-it-alone, nothing's-gonna-hold-me-back-or-

take-me-down, me-versus-the world (or at least me-separate-from-the-world) self-made mentality that is a hallmark of the American way of life—or at least its mythology.

In theory, this sense of political, personal, and economic free will is a liberatory notion, the noble driver of the rugged and rebellious pioneer spirit that mapped the New World and created a cradle of innovation and brought down the tyranny of twentieth-century fascism (while not ignoring, of course, that it also exterminated all the Indigenous who stood in the way and spearheaded the literal and spiritual slaughter of millions of slaves). This sensibility has always been embedded in the cultural coding that runs the behavioral software, despite ideals embedded in pledges and politicians' professions of the opposite—and it proved to be even more true as economic inequality became the norm and not the exception, the basics of life denied to millions of citizens who haven't been "American enough" to earn them. Even when not explicitly espoused, this egoic isolationism is a fundamental underpinning of the "American Way." If it weren't, our infrastructure would include not only freeways and bridges and airports (crumbling though they may be), but also universal health care and subsistence security and easy access to the best education in the world. Maybe these things are coming, finally, to a town near you and near everyone else. (COVID could catalyze this.) Maybe. But the very fact that they haven't been there all along is a telling diagnosis—if not a condemnation—of what America truly values: the individual's (or corporation's) right to transcend without including, to elevate raw power over parity and equity of opportunity for all; the tacit sensibility that economic success equals moral purity, and thus its corollary that penury flows from turpitude or lassitude; and, of course, profit uber alles.

Not to put socialist democracies on a pedestal, but it makes sense that the undergirding of commonality that serves as a foundational social contract in more progressive nations—the belief that access to the necessities of life is a right and not a privilege—builds a scaffolding far different from that of the New World. Buddhism may not be the guiding philosophy Over There, personally or politically, but a sense of inter-being permeates these cultures, is sewn into the very fabric of their societies, while a pronounced lack of engagement in or even acknowledgment of this interconnectedness seems to be a hallmark of the rugged, individualistic "American spirit." (After all, the American Spirit aka Holy Spirit—for, as David Bowie said, God is most surely an American—has given us the Prosperity Gospel, no? The ultimate Good News. For those who are worthy.)

COVID may have banished that illusion of separateness for now, as metaphysical connection is manifested as corporeal transmission—and perhaps the primary revelation of its reign will be an acknowledgment of our interconnected reality. Perhaps a true belief in interconnectedness will become as American as apple pie, baseball, and the military-industrial complex. But if history truly echoes, and if the collective Alzheimer's of the country continues its predominance, likely not. And this individualistic tip of the proverbial iceberg—this feeling that individual rights and "needs" supersede the collective good, that liberty and justice for one trump liberty and justice for all—allows COVID to frolic freely amongst us, more so than anywhere else in the world. (At the time of writing, America is the epicenter of the pandemic.) Of course there are countless exceptions to this rough-hewn "rule," but an entrenched sense of isolationist individualism, of "my personal liberty and freedom first," precludes the commonality of purpose and practice essential to sidelining the coronavirus's transmission (a sidelining that has been so successful in places such as New Zealand and South Korea). Without the unequivocal acknowledgment that, cultural mythology be damned, all of our actions interplay with and affect each other—that, yes, to an extent we are responsible for each other's well-being, or at least should be—even a utilitarian response to such an unprecedented threat is infeasible, let alone a utopian one. As generous and as philanthropic and as fundamentally good as Americans may be individually, the cultural institutions and mythology of the American dream machine do not support a general awareness or valuing of connectivity—unless we're speaking of the digital sense. Individuals are meant to rise above the masses, not the other way around. To believe otherwise is apostasy.

Man cannot live by bread alone, and man cannot live alone alone. But the American Spirit speaks otherwise. It doesn't take a plague to reveal this fundamental flaw in our national character. A myriad of other emergencies may have done the same. But the prolonged crisis of COVID and the cascade of attendant crises it may catalyze (as opposed to the short, sharp shock of 9/11) make it a uniquely singular, if singularly un-amusing, court jester. One who proclaims that not only does the Emperor have no clothes, but also that the one-percent have bought up all the couture, whether high or low, and are saving it for the next plaguey day. Or the next fashion show.

COVID-19 may be a shot across the bow of America the Singular, belying the prevarication of isolated individualism and socio-economic quarantine from each other, the belief that any of us or our actions are truly divorced from those of others in This, Our Increasingly Interconnected World.

Or it could just be a flare in the night, illuminating this one aspect of the mountain of ice as it recedes into the distance, having already left its indelible scar.

2) WORSHIPING THE BERG

The perennial focus, devoid of perennial wisdom, on never-ending economic growth, manifested as the belief that we could and should continue to climb Jacob's Ladder to eternal supply-side paradise, an economic world-without-end as vast and immeasurable as God. All the while ignoring—or refusing to face—the fact that incessant, unchecked growth is exactly what defines an aggressive, obliterative cancer.

Like a slow-motion metastasis, the insatiety of our own perspective and practice and desire consumes us. We tend our homegrown disease and feed it all the nutrients it needs: our beliefs, our actions, our inactions. We catalyze the death wish's growth and thus its devastation not only of our environment but also of our spirit, while ignoring so many other cultural illnesses—and refusing prescriptions for a more healthy, holistic approach to establishing equilibrium for the planet and for the body politic. After a certain tipping point, there is only one end to this carcinogenic path.

The challenge of containing the cancer is exacerbated by the implicit belief that divinity created democracy (and thus capitalism) as part of His divine order, that the stock market and an economic system full of inequity and thus iniquity aren't human choices—that they're as natural and inevitable as the weather used to be, ordained by His Glory and translated into the perfect Platonic form of human fiscal interaction, just as it's "supposed to be." In the American Triumvirate of God, democracy, and the free market, you can't have one without the others because, like the Trinity itself, the three exist not only as individuated realities but also as co-existent and mutually dependent concomitants. Take one out and the whole pyramid (scheme?) falls down. Once you equate divinity with freedom and democracy, and freedom and democracy with unchecked free market capitalism, how can you eradicate or amend the insatiable economic impulse of the hypercapitalist cancer without burning yourself at the stake? God = democracy. Democracy = capitalism (and, even if unintentionally, the cancerous impulse it engenders). Thus, through the transitive property of cultural mores, God = the cancer of capitalism. And God wants you and everyone else to keep building the economic Tower of Babel endlessly upward, the bricks of Mammon mortared by the sweat of labor that, ideally, isn't even yours. According to the "logic" of this largely unquestioned belief system, cancer is as American as Sunday school and ice cream socials. Cancer is what God wants us to have. If you kill the cancer, you kill God. And that heresy can never be. All must worship at the altar of this Great Crab of a Deity, who grows ever more immense and omnipotent through the energy of the worshipers. (As all gods do. Just as they die when there is no one left to sing their praises.) And he who earns the most is, by definition, he who hosannas the loudest.

COVID crept in when we were looking the other way, catalyzing our cancer. Because we have always been looking the other way. Toward the stock market. Or the job market. Or any other arbiter of that Thanatopic impulse toward the ideal of eternally unconstrained growth. When one has cancer, one probably can't think of much else beyond a healing protocol. But when one worships cancer? To fixate on anything else is to abjure God. And thus to lose one's soul.

It doesn't take a COVID-19 to expose the death cult for what it is. Any one of a number of emergencies would do. But this is the crisis we have been "given," a meta-crisis that exposes the underlying crises that have been with us all along. Perhaps it will illuminate the more rational-compassionate notion that limitless economic growth is not always something to be admired or desired, just as we would never cheer on a virus's boundless transmission. (Unless we'd lost our minds, not to mention our souls.) Or, it could make so many want so much More More More—so that enough will still be left, when everything else is gone. So that the ship of the individual is buttressed against any further collective strike.

3) DISASTER ON DEMAND (AND EVERYTHING ELSE, TOO)

The transformation of the country from a congregation of self-sacrifice to a cult of self-indulgence, as the Greatest Generation gave way to the Greatest Commodification—replete with an overarching sense of entitlement, an addiction to instant gratification, a hedonistic impulse that feeds the consumerist cancer, and the idiocratic lack of critical reasoning skills that too often are the natural by-products of our economic drives and our "educational" underpinnings.

Together, these drives constitute a unique sense of American Hubris reinforced by the myth of American Exceptionalism—and reified as American Materialism. We need all that we want, and what we want we assuredly deserve. And that's exactly what we should and will get—that and nothing else. Because surely, through its divine mandate, America the Exceptional cannot get what it does not want. Deadly pandemics? Those are for shit-hole countries. No need to prepare for something we don't even believe in. Good old-fashioned fascism? That's for Europe— and maybe a few other places too. But not here. Not for us.

COVID-19 may correct these courses—at least the materialistic obsessions, as economic resources recede and preclude their possibility. Or it may create a culture in which the have-nots demand their bounty from the haves, the bounty that's been denied them for far too long through stacked decks and tilted chess boards. In a culture of community and commonality, man vs. man conflict would be constrained, alchemically transformed into man vs. the common "invisible enemy." Because, after all, in reality there is plenty to go around. But American mythology precludes beliefs that belie the materialistic zero-sum game. It refuses to acknowledge that all boats can be lifted, regardless of the nature of the tide, and instead allows too many to list and lurch as they try to keep their occupants' heads above water.

Three layers of the cultureware coalesced into the perfect iceberg, the one that could take down the ostensibly impervious ship of state: the mythology of individualism and thus disconnection from any sense of responsibility for the Other—or at least for the Others that exist outside one's own tribe; the manifest destiny of eternal economic expansion and the worship of a "divinely mandated" cancer as an end unto itself, as opposed to seeing economic systems as a human and necessarily curtailable means to a healthier homeostasis—medically, economically, educationally, ecologically, and even existentially; a self-centered, self-absorbed, hubristic credo of convenience, indulgence, and invulnerability, a system that shackles us to wants rather than needs—while, through the starved and strangled corpse of our educational system, delimiting the type of rational contemplation that would clarify the folly of it all.

Titanic Nation. Self-actuated iceberg struck. The ship would have sunk, eventually, even without the exacerbating influence of these plague days, a victim of its own unwieldy weight and untenable appetites. (And no one is saying that this virus is the Beginning of the End of American Empire, economically and thus otherwise. While it very well may be.) COVID-19 has merely put everything in stark relief.

While COVID-19 is not the iceberg, it's an easy scapegoat for what ails us. A fictive bogeyman to blame for systemic shortcomings that are now coming to the fore, particularly economically—the consequences of which may make the medical exigencies little more than the opening act. (To externalize our own shortcomings and project them onto an outside influence may be all-too-human but, of course, this impulse merely prolongs the problem.) The virus is not the iceberg. Nor did it break the berg from its glacial sheath. All of that happened long ago, independent of virological influence. But This Thing seems uniquely engineered to exploit the characteristics of the cultureware that runs the system that built this particular ship—and thus created all its attendant vulnerabilities. All nations' states will be degraded under COVID's auspices, when the Before COVID calendar is compared with the After Destabilization era. But perhaps none more so than the Titanic's. (And note that the use of the word *engineered* is not to suggest that COVID-19 is some sort of orchestrated bio-attack or black op. While neither option is beyond the pale, both conspiracy theories and politics are as useful here as a band-aid on a decapitation.)

COVID-19 simply Is, and its Isness is incontrovertible. Where it came from is not the point. Where it leads us Is.

As to that leading . . . as to why there's no reason for (or allowing of) wailing on the decks of the ship: that is the true lesson of these, our challenging plague days. Even if the ship is sinking—and yes that's an "if" since, like nautical technology, economic and medical technocracies have evolved since the literal iceberg strike of a century ago, and our psychospiritual bilges are more capacious than ever—there is no reason for despair. Or submission. (While an element of fear, unfortunately, will be with anyone who is paying attention. Fear is fine. Cowardice is not.)

If the greatest nautical wonder of the early twentieth century can be capsized, then the iceberg too can be inverted, making the imminence and eminence of its threat impossible to ignore any longer. And through that inversion, we can embrace the opposites of its layers of self-destruction. We can flip our Shiva instincts on their heads, taking the insanity of our topsy-turvy ways and settling them right-side up in the land of the sane. And even if it's too late to fully right the wrongs and thus salvage the ship, we can ensure the greatest survival rate, physically and psychically, by slowing the sinking so there is time to create the rescue plan we so desperately need.

Because unlike the historical disaster, there are lifeboats aplenty— as long as we don't get distracted by a siren song emanating from deep within the ice, calling us back to old ways and archaic attitudes that are no longer seaworthy.

By suggesting that we board those lifeboats, by exploring what we have to gain from the challenge of our context, I do not intend to trivialize the coronavirus catastrophe. While a College of COVID may exist, in that this experience has much to teach us individually and collectively (as all experiences do, no matter how triumphant or traumatic), you'll find no act of dismissive optimism here through which, unwittingly even, victims are blamed and the wreckage is worshiped. This is not some disaster utopianist screed about how we all deserved 9/11 because of this nation's political sins and that maybe our national karma could finally be reset. That the catastrophe of the Iraq War was recompense for a self-indulgent society hopped up on its own sense of entitlement and invulnerability. Or that COVID is a "good thing." What was "meant to be."

While most people appreciate—or are at least enthralled by—a good old-fashioned shipwreck, on the circumference of mainstream thought there lies a type of nascent jubilation regarding our current virological conundrum: a feeling that COVID is what had to happen, that it's a critical message from Mama Gaia and damn it maybe now we'll finally listen, and surely it's all worth it even if millions have to die (because isn't it about time, as Ebenezer Scrooge said, "to decrease the surplus population"?)—not to mention the countless multitudes who have suffered and who will suffer due to the potential economic apocalypse—because All of Them (but certainly not All of Us) are just the collateral damage of a great rebirthing, right? And the collective mass of all those struggling souls is like a vanishing twin who dies in utero so that its sibling can absorb all its life, but it will all be fine in the end because, after all, I've been preparing for this my whole life—well, maybe not preparing per se, but I went to the right school and got the right socially distant job and now, while I may not be immune to the virus, I'm immune to the context that makes contracting the virus more likely and so, while my social world may have shrunk, my economic and subsistence existence is doing just fine, thank you very much—and if This is What Is, then its Is-Ness must be What Must Be, What Should Be, and when the dust settles and the pathogen pisses off it will all be hunky-dory (at least for me and mine) because, after all, we've needed this kind of reboot for a long time. The Earth is speaking! The Divine Mind is transmitting and making itself manifest here in Malkuth, the miraculous media of burning bushes and plagues of locusts elegantly translated into microscopic, scientific materialistic terms that make sense to the postmodern mind.

(Excuse the hyperbole, but there's been too much of this talk, if not so overt—primarily from New Agey upper-ish echelons of the socio-economic food chain, those who can most ride out the churning waters until some semblance of calm rolls through, an internal wave that brings at least an interregnum of "peace" or "normalcy." It feels like a uniquely capitalist, rugged individualistic stance of "I got mine," devoid of the undergirding of empathy and sense of inter-being that we need to ride This Thing out in the most humane manner possible. Like the protagonist in Lars von Trier's *The Five Obstructions* banqueting amidst starving children in the slums of Mumbai, a certain kind of sensibility is able to sit easy with the carnage and dance on the tombstones. Some would say this stance is heartless in its lack of empathy. Others may claim it's enlightened in its transpersonal transcendence of individual ego boundaries and needs, all for the "greater glory." Regardless, the world is drowning in the fluid of its own lungs. And the ship of state sputters on, wondering when it can dock back home where it came from—while knowing, consciously or not, it never can. Because that home no longer exists, and likely never will. Because it never really did.)

Yes, silver (or at least copper) linings may exist. In the psychospiritual stuff of COVID's structure we may find a potential to rebirth ourselves into a more harmonious relationship with Earth and each other. But the three layers of the iceberg have created a culture that, when the ship begins to sink, is less able to engage unity and more likely to embrace entropy.

Extrinsic adversaries are much easier to vanquish. But when the enemy is ourselves? All else—whether war or plague or famine or any other horseman to come clopping along—is just an onrush of ocean waves filling the bilge whose pumps have already gone bad. All else merely exploits the weaknesses already extant in the hubristic, individualistic, carcinogenic hull of Titanic Us.

COVID-19 is the messenger of our great disconnect, from each other and from what we should truly value, if we wish the grasp of our worldly walk to match the reach of our foundational talk. COVID-19 is the ship crier shouting out that the vessel has been struck while too many of us were partying below deck, unaware of the unfolding tragedy because we were too distracted by the great frolic. What was invisible or unimportant for so many is now manifest for all to see. But COVID alone could never prey upon us in a way that leads to decimation. It's merely the crisis that underscores the self-made predatory crises that were already swimming below the surface—and potentially swells them to an untenable size.

So now we have a meta-crisis, a crisis that speaks of and exposes all the other cultural calamities. (Had it not been COVID it would have been something else. Another senseless war. Another economic implosion and the unrest it could cause. Or something else theoretically obvious but practically unimaginable, as COVID was to the mainstream mind. A terminal cancer can manifest in many ways, can claim many different organs. But the end game is the same, despite the particularities of the manifestation.) A disease in and of itself, COVID is also a symptom of the underlying ailments that can cause disastrous collapse. It is the revelation of the undercurrent of cultural crisis, the John the Baptist of the illness in our systemic beliefs and actions that lead not to messianic salvation but to auto-executed damnation. The dis-eases were always there. But now they are impossible to ignore.

And so: the powers-that-be never let a good crisis go to waste. And neither should "we." It may not seem there are enough lifeboats to go around. But certainly there are. For all women. All children. And all men.

As to the nature of those lifeboats? Simple enough. They are the antitheses of the elements of the berg that's struck. Community rather than competition (or at least a good-sportsman-like sense of competition, whereby the ingenuity and inspiration it engenders create a mutually beneficial context, a more transcendent expression of this American impulse that, admittedly, used to serve the country well). Interbeing as opposed to isolationist individualism (or at least a hyper-conscious insistence on balance between the two, never abandoning the rebellious soul that birthed the nation but never allowing it to run roughshod over the awareness of others). The love of Enough instead of lusting after Never Enough (with humility reigning over hubris, need over want, gratitude over gratification, Knowing over mere knowledge).

To believe that Titanic Nation can learn a new course may seem an irrational hope. But we are still a young dog of a nation. And sanity should never be measured by "reasonableness" as measured by a dominant cultural paradigm that is patently insane. We may be adrift, the iceberg struck and others likely lurking beyond the horizon (at least while glaciers still exist). We may be cruising through frigid and frightening waters swimming with a multitude of invisible predators, ready to exploit our self-inflicted wounds. An inordinate number of passengers could perish, or at least be imperiled. Or the vast majority could survive, and maybe even thrive. We must do what we always should, whether in times of trouble or transcendence: elevate ourselves and our circles (while always trying to expand both their area and circumference), with the ultimate aim of elevating the world. The transformations we undertake will carry us through turbulence. And when calm descends, they will make the peace even more prosperous. Repairing the hull is simple in theory. As for practice: it can be hard to push against a monstrous tide.

And even if a sinking is inevitable, if it's what the cosmos "commands" or if it's too late because the damage is beyond any reparation, there is neither need nor time to indulge in nihilistic despair. We can still choose, as always, to make the sinking as grace-full as it can be. As compassionate and connected and kind as the songs of our higher angels can sing.

The great journey down can be barbaric or benevolent; in an America acculturated to competition rather than collaboration, it can seem panacea-ic to believe in the eventuality of the latter rather than the former. Were it not for the iceberg we made, we have (and have always had) the resilience and the resources to "easily" rectify all our woes, both pre-COVID and post, through the collaborative co-creation of new paradigms, perspectives, and practices. But in competition the iceberg allows these distressors not only to exist but to endlessly express like those metastatic cells. We've been divided as a nation since the day we were born (maybe even before, if the soul of America is but the reincarnation of an earlier empire). And the truth is, COVID won't get us. Only we can get ourselves. In the most destructive sense imaginable. Or in the most transcendent future imagined.

COVID is not the cure for what ails us. But it could be the coronation of a greater consciousness that before was only an ideal. But which now is exigency.

◆ ◆ ◆

Like the infamous iceberg it is not, COVID-19 may feel cataclysmic. And climactic. In reality, medically and economically, it's only just begun. Whether the first act of a greater script or warm-up for a more vicious virological routine or a warning of the shape of things to come, this is the prelude to what can feel like the nocturne of our lives. And it's not over until a "final" song is sung. To some extent, it's a song we've all been waiting for, stuck on our respective ships of state all around the world. (Some ships are just better at riding the waves.)

Regardless of whether we can self-rescue as effectively as we've self-disconnected—or the extent to which we can—COVID no longer lets anyone believe that the Ship of American State is still seaworthy. It tells us that it's time to embrace the All Connection and eschew the illusory sense of separateness that can transform a miraculous vessel into a ghost ship. It's time to kill the cancer as much as we want to immunize against the insidious virus. It's time to start patching the hull, while the violins play above deck. And—whether through some act of providence or collective and concentrated human-ness—it's time to experience the rising of the tide that lifts everyone up.

Let the sirens sing their song of allurement and destruction. And let us avoid their call, swaying to a less titanic tune, dancing and singing with the violins if we have to go down, communing with each other all the way—while knowing we can still save the ship and thus ourselves. If only we sing our own song instead.

Eric Myers splits his time between San Francisco and Columbus, Ohio, writing and teaching from the Haight and from his book bunker in the Short North. A playwright in remission, he is the cofounder of MADLAB in Ohio and Burning Man Information Radio in California. His latest act of "conceptual architecture" is the Biblioteca Esoterica, a private membership library and underground arts space in Columbus that specializes in rare and out-of-print editions. He can be contacted at eric@ericmyers.net.

AGAINST AN ENDEMIC RESPONSE

Robert Podgurski

Nothing on earth has a right to live, only a chance, a chance.
—Jim Trainor, *The Moschops*, 2000

Responding in writing to the worldwide event known as the COVID-19 epidemic is subject to an infinite number of variables. Working toward a *best response* may perhaps be as allusive an endeavor as attempting to respond medically to the virus itself. *Allusive* was actually a typo whereas I intended *elusive,* but I left this perceived mistake in place as proof in the pudding of the grand aporia that appears to be taking place right now as a result of the contagion. And by aporia I am implying an empuzzlement, a quandary that somehow resides outside all accepted modes of cognition. Making this assertion is and is not a rhetorical maneuver on my part. I am attempting to logically address the disease, what it ultimately pertains to and represents, as something operating with a purpose that supersedes all hominid-based rationale. Many have suggested that mankind's evolution is the result of a viral mutation, and some have even gone so far as to suggest that we as a race have evolved from a virus itself. Adhering to that line of reasoning may compel one to formulate that COVID-19 is a building block in man's evolution; it may very well be. Or it could be the opposite. Or even more thought-provoking: it could be both—evolution and devolution. This apophasis, and now we're dealing partly with the rhetorical component of said aporia, may allude to the possibility of COVID-19 acting as a sort of *Pharmakon,* or that which kills as it heals. However, I am not so much concerned with positing that the virus may be endowed with this specific variable purpose as I am interested in considering that it may be an embodiment of a contradictory nature that *eludes* all standard reasoning.

Salomo Friedlaender in his seminal work, *Der Schöpferische Indifferenz,* or *Creative Indifference,* asserted that there exists a grey area between darkness and light, hot and cold, life and death—that is not discernable in ordinary terms. It is a space where ground, background, and foreground dissolve into one another. And it is in this space of dissolution that boundaries become naught, where the force of pure creative inception resides, ultimately there for the making.

Allowing for such a possibility hints at a viral organism whose ultimate purpose or implications may evade all current attempts to denote. Perhaps, at a future time the condition and end-result of this epidemic and all of its side-effects will provide us with a qualifying perspective of the overall significance.

But for now, it spreads. And I have purposefully avoided referring to this virus as a *pan*demic because I tend to be very literal about nomenclature. *Pandemia* would suggest, at least to me, a condition whose bounds exceed known ones including humanity. That is why I used *endemic* in the title. I am not just addressing the condition of contagion as one specific to mankind but the notion itself as such. I'm not ready to utilize the term *pandemic* in its literal and expanded sense to address this current global health crisis and all that it encompasses. It has not had an opportunity to work its way through and out of our dated perspective. If it weren't dated, then the Black Death, the Spanish flu of 1918, and other global scourges would tell us all we need to know and we'd have it figured out. Rather, the tale is being retold, which makes me think of Husserl's statement that a story within a story is not actually a story but a *re*-presentation of one. The current mode of explanations offered via the media and governmental organizations is very similar to internal dialogue, propagated in an attempt to keep one and all from going crazy. Otherwise, in the face of facts, silence would be welcome. But it never is.

The un-reasoning effect that all emergencies have on people is well known and pronounced. If COVID-19 eventually elicits a rejection of the norm—the accepted logic in perceiving how widespread illness factors into our biocentricity, behavior, and possibly spirituality—then it would mean that learning has taken place. The in-betweenness or creatively indifferent realm that this specific virus catalyzes within the commonly understood polarities of health and illness would then hit a plateau. I think of a previously unrealized bodhisattvic condition, one that is born of a new epoch, but that's only due to my modernist leanings and deficiencies that derive from a dependence on historicity. Ideally, an extinction of the ever-narrowing confines of ideology and dogma will be the only viral response we'll be confronting in the near future.

Robert Podgurski has been practicing magick, qi gong, and yoga for over thirty years. His occult investigations have formed the basis of his monograph on the practical applications of extra-dimensional sigils, *The Sacred Alignments and Sigils*. A second edition was released by North Atlantic Books in 2019. This monograph explores the complex relationships among sigils, John Dee's Enochian magick, telluric influences, and the corporeal. Podgurski is currently at work on Part Two, *The Aetheric Alignments*. He has been lecturing on sigils, magick, and the occult influence in poetry for over thirty years. His poetry collection *Wandering on Course* was released by Spuytin Duyvil Press in 2014.

MAKE THIS TIME COUNT

Kristina Joy Gutiérrez

Breathing deeply is not canceled.

Being kissed by the sun is not canceled.

Feeling grateful to be alive is not canceled.

Singing, playing music, dancing is not canceled.

Creating a new and better version of ourselves is not canceled.

Emanating positive vibes to the planet is not canceled.

Having hope is not canceled.

Being present, here and now, is not canceled.

Loving one another is not canceled.

Letting go of what no longer serves us is not canceled.

Forgiveness is not canceled.

Inner Freedom from mental slavery is not canceled.

Starting over, as many times as we need to, is not canceled.

We are not dead yet.

So LIVE. And make the time that we have been blessed with count.

April 1, 2020

KRISTINA JOY is a vibrational resonance sound therapist, energy healing practitioner, breathwork facilitator, meditation teacher, certified life coach, and artist with a master's in education. She strongly believes in the notion that when we heal ourselves, we heal the world, because peace worldwide starts from inside. Kristina Joy's mission is to help as many people as she can to achieve inner peace, deep healing, true happiness, an awakening of consciousness, and a sense of oneness with everyone and everything.

BODY HEAT

Lindy Hough

The state of California is in quarantine.
Shelter-at-home feels like house arrest.
If you *have* your mask on a walk,
that's good enough, don't need to wear it. But
that stymies the point of a mask: to shield others
from your unintentional flying droplets
and be shielded from others' trajectories.

Encountering a pedestrian
I take big half circles
into the street, hardly any cars anyway,
greeting strangers warmly, if shyly.
I relate to people walking home
from Berkeley much more than
before the pandemic.

How did it start?
At first we thought someone
ate a bat carrying the virus
in Wuhan, China.
But that ends up blaming China.
Blame is not the same as

fact: I can state fact w/o meaning
blame. Is that not true? There's been
no other received explanation.
We have good intel on this.

POTUS blames China. He takes a smidgen of fact
and twists it to suggest he discovered this,
a dagger to hurt, in this case a country.

We know from the SARS virus that the coronavirus
originates in bats. *The only mammal adapted for
flight.* A bat's body temperature soars
to 108°F while flying, its tiny heart thumps
like fast staccato, rising to 1,000 beats per minute.

Bats are creatures with very sharp teeth who
come out only at night, seeing by sound.

Eating dinner outdoors, my family
used to watch bats at dusk,
recognizing them as different from
birds by their jagged prowl.

The balance of their hot body and
fast heartbeat gives bats an ideal internal
climate, providing a defensive
tolerance for viruses living in them
peacefully.

It's not bats. It's what we do with bats
that loads this pandemic risk.

And what do we do? We eat them raw.

Did a SuperCarrier catch
COVID-19 from eating a raw
bat? How many people and how many bats?

Many diseased carrier bats? Or was just one
bat with the virus biting one person
enough to cause this?

What will we learn from this?
Impermanence. Yes, everything changes.
Dragonflies. Monarch butterflies. Milkweed.

LINDY HOUGH is a poet and fiction writer. She is the author of five books of
poetry: *Changing Woman, Psyche, The Sun in Cancer, Outlands & Inlands,* and
Wild Horses, Wild Dreams: New and Selected Poems 1971–2010. She has com-
pleted a novel about a Denver family during the uranium boom in the Four
Corners area in the early 1950s. She lives in Berkeley, California, and Portland,
Maine. www.lindyhough.com.

PRAYERS FOR CORONA

Vicki Robin

Nightly prayers

Now I lay me down to sleep
I pray the lord my soul to keep
And if the virus take my life
I pray the lord to send me right
Back as a sturgeon full of eggs
Or as a milkweed blowing seeds
Or as a bear that births twins and twins again
That feed on salmon on their long last swim
Past concrete icebergs of dams now gone
Heading home like me, to feed my ones
Now I lay me down to sleep
I pray my soul the bees to keep
Oh let me be a queen engorged with young
And let the blossoms feed my sons
And let the fruit drop to the ground
And let the worms feast long and sound
Like nectar to mycelia, hidden down.
Oh let the earth come back alive
The swarming birds the buzzing hive
And let trees drink in what I breathe out.

Let their roots feed on me as I rot.
Oh let my cells run off my bones
To feed my mother, to feed my home.
Now we lay us down to sleep
We pray the lord to find us here
Her children once again made whole
We pray he breathes our singing souls.

RIGHT AT LAST

Hail Mary full of grace
Be with us now and in the hour of our deaths
The Mary Maria and Marlene
who've died this week of Corona, the crown.
And Joseph and Giuseppe and Joe
And Tom and Lisa and Susan and more
We need to say the names of those
Who've passed as the virus claims our loves
Yuri, Sadie, Adam and Eve
Gone through virus gone to their graves
Say Kaddish for all we cannot name
Sam and Lucy and Manu and Lam
How many names have not been said
how strong the dread how many dead
Kim and Kuri and Peggy and Jen
Curt and Alvin and Mike and more not said
The dead of corona, the dead of attacks
Of hearts and livers and dengue and cars
Holy Mary Mother of God and Godfrey and Geoff and Rod
Pray for us now and in the hour of our deaths
For we have sinned and we have loved
Pray for us
Pray for the praying mantis
Pray for all children of all species for all time

Pray for all who die and pray for all who live
May we release them from their grief
And let them travel on.
Let our dreams die with us and be reborn
In someone else, yet to come
Hail Mary Maria Marlene
Ave Maria
Ave Maria
Hail this Crown full of grace.

VICKI ROBIN, coauthor of *Your Money or Your Life* and of *Blessing the Hands that Feed Us,* is a longtime writer, speaker, and social innovator on issues of resilience, resourcefulness, climate limits, and simplicity. She blogs at http://vickirobin.com.

THE CENTER OF THE WORLD IS CHANGING LOCATION

Rob Brezsny

Last night I dreamed that I had caught the virus. It hadn't made me sick. My body felt stronger than usual—and much denser; as if I were on a planet with greater gravitational pull.

So the invading presence, the virus, wasn't causing disease, but was rather like a psychedelic drug that had flooded my consciousness with five additional levels of awareness. Three of the new layers were dark and two were luminous. At times I imagined myself as a bioluminescent marine creature floating languidly near the ocean's bottom.

The virus had possessed me from both the inside and the outside. I was under its spell. It wasn't an unpleasant feeling, but neither was it pleasant; not light or sweet or "fun," but very demanding and consuming. I was grateful for the chance to raise my courage in response to its relentless teachings.

On several occasions, I addressed it as if it were a sentient being.

"Are you friend or foe?" I asked it.

"Neither and both," it said—not with a voice but like a text-message coalescing in the blood flowing to my heart from my right arm.

"You feel so heavy inside me," I said. "Like lead made from gold."

"Why don't you gladly and completely empty yourself of your thoughts about who I was, am, and will be?" it replied.

"Is it OK if I make jokes about you?" I said.

"Do you think I have no soul?" it said, in what seemed like a laugh.

Some of the virus's teachings came in the form of riddles. "Where did you live before you lived everywhere?" was one. My answer: "I lived nowhere."

Another riddle it posed: "When you figure out how to change me as much as I change you, you'll be me and I'll be you. We'll be dangerously safe together."

"I'll be a lover-warrior fighting and adoring you," I said.

The dream was the longest dream I ever recall having. It flowed on for many days and nights, although even the days were shadowy twilight. I never traveled anywhere, but mostly writhed and rolled around on warm ground. Sometimes I lay still and shivered with whatever the opposite of the chills are.

To succeed at my initiation—and it did feel like an initiation administered by remote tribal elders working in concert with the virus, as if they and the virus were linked by radio waves—I had to work very hard to keep monitoring and registering the new ways of understanding reality that were surging into my awareness. The new understandings ran the gamut between PARADISE IS NOWHERE and PARADISE IS NOW HERE.

I periodically told myself, "Stay awake and alert as you live through this ceremony of transformation."

A certain feminine elder I respected—a blend of Rebecca Solnit and Naomi Klein—appeared now and then to offer comments and support. Near the end of the ordeal, she said, "The center of the world is changing location."

Rob Brezsny writes the internationally syndicated column "Free Will Astrology" and is the author of the book *Pronoia Is the Antidote for Paranoia: How the Whole World Is Conspiring to Shower You with Blessings.* His website is FreeWillAstrology.com.

PORTAL POEMS

Zoe Brezsny

Untitled

can you see the row of lights
vibrating from crescent city

floating in the air / hanging by a thread

before the century

stimulus key turned

in pleasure
then thrown into the game's sexless sky

cash in on

demon claws

you and me as inanimate objects

safeway chocolate chip cookies

pesticides mixed
quietly with essential nutrients

tip toe past

periphery of a collective hallucination

FREE Mood

and Depression Screener

calcified blind spots
form mosaic patterns

What's inside you what's
looking in

for critical cellular data

If I am approved,
How do I claim it?

tear swept
Earth

salt lick

The kitten pulls on her belly button ring in the dimly lit room

watched from afar

Eye to Eye Delirium
After Sofia Sinibaldi

What's a scam and what's for real

lactic acidosis and gut feelings

my twin flame

reddit subthreads predict

molten tears down clown cheeks

ways of seeing in the dark

scan
a thousand years marked on a tree

the size of the eyes
between a cherry and a walnut

A humming swarm maps
a surrounding environment

mineral reservoirs

my reward system

visions of a new world

a coded pattern left in a driveway

dayglo X

hot concrete in the empty street

my invisible friends
warm and wet behind the eyes

Face filter *Yourlove2020*

Violation #83817543

Microsoft asks where do you want to go today

Love scene in the sea

Anxiety washed over by the moonlight

the grit of salt

a pure love

fucking the ocean

twilight series on the plane

portals to other places in the universe

Time square Olive Garden

A celebrity named reality winner

A sacred site
in a rental car parking lot

Soft bank promises to build
a more connected, efficient,
joyful world

Humanity has been following a program for millions of years

The universe is infinite which means
there are infinite possibilities

simultaneously knowing
this while depressed

You shine in the body
The sun shines deeper than thought

I see friends coming out of drug stores
And want to tell them their hidden talents
not so hidden at all
just by the society we live in
they can't see them

doesn't matter in five years
doesn't matter

There's only love and fear

A fountain flows on Seneca Avenue

I forgot
the sensual breeze
of the veil blowing across
lifting my depression

ZOE BREZSNY is a poet and organizer who lives in New York. She curated
Parallax, a reading series of contemporary poetry at Hauser & Wirth Gallery.
She co-runs the project space Gern en Regalia in the Lower East Side. Listen to
archives of her radio show at wfmu.org.

AT THE EDGE OF THE GREAT SWAMP
Seven Poems of Redemption Midst the Virus

Paul Weiss

Starting

If we must start somewhere,
let's start with mist.
Let's start with this gray first morning
of spring; a clock ticking; a crow.
Let's start with that brush pile,
waiting to be burned before the rain
begins; this warm sip of tea; this
breath; this burp. Let's appreciate the
way life has been scattered like
pick-up sticks, shifting like dreams.
Enjoy the array. No hurry.
Soon you will act.

Gone Viral

I finally got it. Just sit
and do anything. Ponder. Stare. Wander
around the house; pick up a
magazine. Put it down. I walk in
my woods. I rake last year's leaves.

Those are the peaks.

Late afternoon, I sit by the window.
Watch this light snow, so modest
and discreet. It's the 30th of March;
and it's been a gentle season so
we have only good will for
these innocent snowflakes,
skipping like schoolyard children
this way and that. Keeping a
social distance from each other.
Refusing to stick. They have gotten
the message. We are all pulling
together to stay apart. Stay put; keep
moving. Don't visit. Don't cling.

Don't work. But find something meaningful. Ah, that's the trap
of an earnest mind. The world is
under siege, and out of joint. Be useful,
be fruitful. Surely my strong point;
but no. I wander in circles. I hide
my naked restlessness under the ragged
cloak of occasional relevance;
wisdom; service; art. I look at the sky;
or frown. I pick up a book on trees.
Or put it down. Things fall apart.
I hear the radio: the clues.

This time I get it! There is only one
news and it includes all news.
The news is everywhere. Just find a
chair. Or find a snack. Distract
yourself. Walk on the road. Rake last
year's leaves. Let time go down

the drain. It is a good drain. It is
the drain by which things enter and
things leave. Or care. Or are released.
Or bask in unknown relevance.
Or sit in peace. Or stare.

MARCH 30, 2020

WOULD YOU SIT WITH ME THAT SLOW?

When the focus is still,
you can see the moon move
higher above the treetops.

The slower you sit,
the faster the moon moves;

As fast as the tide
rising on a quiet bay.

Can you feel the ache
for a home when the earth
was that slow?

And you could hear the breeze
inviting each needle of the fir
to dance in the moonlight.

When watching the moon rise
was the only news—and to watch
was our only ambition.

When life was analogue, and the brain
fired like a slow leaping dancer
over the fields of light,

and the moon-stirred waters
of the black sky
settled under the skin.

Would you sit with me that slow,

like someone who had the time
to put his money
on the winning snail?

Spring Morning

Dampness rises from the morning earth.
Smoke from the fire.
The body growls a bit and sends out its warmth too.
Rain in the air. The trees know everything.
Thoughts, feelings: it's all snow melt.
This growling is a subterranean hum. Let's growl along.
Something complete is moving as the earth moves.
Resting on our foundation, the universe is accomplished.
Heart recognizing heart. The rest is artifact.
Didn't we pass this way a million years from now?
I'm gonna let this timeless buggy take us home;
stick with what's true; sing with the clacking wheels.
Simple opportunity is given every day—
which we cast out with the morning sink water.
Trying to manage the world by thought is
like trying to balance a cup atop a gushing fountain;
or to operate the sunrise from a smartphone.
I think I'll let the day play me for a fool.
Be just as stupid as this rainfall.
Give me a ring, and we'll walk together.

At the Edge of the Great Marsh

On the late afternoon marsh, a sea of reed grass
trembles in the least breeze.

This is the pregnant hush of a great voice.
This is the language of the slow.

Here in the awake world is a mutual respect.
The grasses and their witness

are of one intelligence.
The mosquitos nod and give safe passage.

We are each of the other.
Only this silent . . . hearing begins.

Only this slow . . . the earth moves.
There is no forbidden door,

but we do not seek admittance;
we do not bow in entry before the great open.

There is a community as vast and intimate
as space, and we are its lost children.

I have come back to my home
by the great pine at the edge of the great marsh.

Lone spider threads glisten silver in the late sun
like slender streaks of moonlight.

All share one tremulous anticipation as sun paints
the marsh from descending angles,

and the air grows cool: The Great Mother Bear
is coming in her dark robes

to hold close the trembling tribes;
to wear them as her own fur.

To keep them to the world's end.
To be shown through with the new day.

RADIO FREE PLEASURE

There is hope for us here,
beyond the barbed wire fences of the mind,
the propaganda of its loudspeakers
squawking its old sad tune; its message of
need and lack. Unseen behind the old tool shed,
we sit and tune our dials to the thin band
of attention and surrender ready to receive the
ever growing voice from the world beyond
the Camp; beyond the stifling oppression
of the guards, and our poor found substitutes
for joy or freedom.

It is our hard won faithfulness to keeping
the dial tuned that welcomes in a growing stream
of good news, a growing clarity and lightness.
Until, through the static, we pick up the signal of a
steady stream of pleasure, beamed from we know
not where, beamed at no cost, no monthly plan.
It is a pleasure unconstructed and unsought for,
taking over our bodies, inviting us to the next level
of discernment; the next release.

When we look again, the barbed wire is melting,
the loudspeakers silenced; the guards are puppy dogs.
Casually, we pull others aside, one by one,
from their mindless collaboration with the work gangs,
the death squads; and slip the earphones over their
heads, tune the dial, sit still, and watch their growing
smiles, as slowly they discern the silent voice
of Radio Free Pleasure.

GREAT HEAD

(FOR ADAM)

1.

Walking the shoreline, kicking wet sand
from my shoes, following the path your soul
might have traveled to release itself
from your body. I ascend the higher rocks.
Could it have been here, or here, where you entered
the water? And there where the currents might
have carried you after several days? Your
soul like a lemon twist added to these waters;
wrung out, twisted; all these lemons, only
you couldn't make lemonade. The rowboat
wasn't steady, although all the fresh ingredients
were yours at the start. When the wolves were quiet,
the mud slides cleared away, a true fire gleamed
from the inner cave. Your journey is ours.

2.

It is a privilege to witness this late afternoon sparkle
of sun on the ocean. The late breeze
not knowing whether to blow warm or cold.
Spring like a toddler trying to find her balance on the
paths out of winter. Even the inevitable is brave.

It is a secret joy to be the raw energy of life,
the outlawed *id* of divine pedigree. To feel the thrill
of radiant being under the fingernails; to feel the
truest skin under the skin of our misgivings,
never going into exile with the mind's self-exile,
but singing consistently in the branches
outside our prison gate, cooing "Touch me, I am
already yours." Touch me even in the moods

of your bleakest winds; find me in the motions of
your mundane tasks; feel me in the respirations
of the heart, whose pleasure is your only currency.

3.
It is a privilege to mourn. To savor the gift
of frailty at the peak of each wave—collapsing as
it goes. And to pause and to kick here against
the driftwood and the bladderwrack with our stubborn
humanity. To walk in the company of a world
so vulnerable that its very appearance is the promise
of its passing; while where it has come from, and where
it has gone, is a space more real than the object
we tried to grasp. It is a delicate proposition, this
body-mind with so many moving parts, each so capable
of dent, tangle, or recoil; each so capable of bleeding
in a world so creative in its pain. It is a privilege
to grieve; and so concede, not in defeat, to the dark roots
of our own breathing; to the incessant breeze
against this shore; to the wind that will carry us
as a dry leaf to its sunlit rest.

A poet since childhood, PAUL WEISS has spent most of his adult life on the coast of Maine. He began his study of zen and tai chi in New York in the mid-sixties, and continued his studies in India and China over the course of many years. He founded The Whole Health Center in Bar Harbor in 1981 as a vehicle for his teaching, counseling, meditation retreats, and healing work, evolving a Buddhist and *tonglen*-based therapeutic model of compassion, integration, and healing. He is the author of *You Hold This,* a book of poems, and *Moonlight Leaning Against an Old Rail Fence—Approaching the Dharma as Poetry,* a collection of poems and commentaries.

A DOZEN POEMS IN THE TIME OF COVID

James Moore

Contagion

Contagion rolls out across the lands
and over the seas
it rides the air
as it jumps the moats of our resistance
scattering the aware before it
consuming the complacent within it
like a spark that starts to spread
a slow burn destroying before it touches
all we hold dear and safe.
Somewhere an old archetype of the apocalypse rides
dryly coughing as it rises to embrace us all
in one of those rare moments
that defines not just a year, or a generation or a life,
but an age when so much is lost so fast
and yet, so much found
of the simple values
we moderns have forgot.

LIFE IN THE TIME OF COVID

This is the end of fun boy, but it's only begun,
opening credits still rolling and the death knell not done
it's all just so sad, everyone huddled inside
alone with their internet on a strange kind of ride
when along comes the trickster as a coyote or crow
to tap on your window and say "Time to go!"
but go where it don't tell us as we walk through the wall
and on down the street right into a mall
where the shops are all empty not an item to buy
'cause the ones there before us were too scared to die
but the brave and the foolish have no fear of death
it's the place we all go when we run out of breath
as our lungs fill with fluid and our minds clog with fear
when we step through THAT wall Death is closer than near
closer than heart beats, and swifter than thought
it's the face in the mirror when at last we are caught
between a rock and a hard place or so it does seem,
till that too breaks open and we see it's a dream
the same one as always, the same as it's been
with Death on our shoulder His face in a grin
as seers watch from cliff sides points of light in their caves
we ride on a tide, the crest of a knave
of the one who has sown fear, lies and deceit
the smart who control all with their ways of conceit
the idea that they know what is beyond grasp
the taste of a lover, or the bite of an asp
the soft sound of silence, or the color of soul
the age of an infant, or the shape of a whole
these things we can ponder but never will know
despite what they tells us, despite what they show
while the pug in his wisdom is so full of joy
at the fountain of youth he's such a good boy

no end of fun for the likes of that dog
it's onward and upward and out through fog . . .

Beyond Fear

What is on the other side . . .
what is when all is let go
when fear is passed through
and we let it just flow
to a shore with wet sands
to a hilltop's broad view
to a bed that is warm
with a love that is true?
What is discovered when all is let go
is it a world of our making
or one we don't know?
Is it a place of our horrors
or a field of our dreams
or is it something beyond
something we thought it would seem?
When we let go of fear
with wide open arms
will the world hug us back
revealing her charms,
or will we stand all alone
rejected by none
but free, free at last
to shine in the sun.

Leave No Trace

Step into nothingness
my little one
let the Great Night swallow you whole
be a spark

be a fire
that gently burns away
to leave no trace
when the morning comes.

WITH LIGHT

I walked through the market
but there was nothing I wanted to buy,
nothing I thought I needed,
until the smile
on the faces of a few
gave me what can't be bought,
and in that moment I drained the full cup
I'd been carefully holding,
and filled it anew
with light.

CREATIVE DESTRUCTION

Life is an endless creative unfolding
each moment giving rise to the next
only by its absolute sacrifice.
So it's ironic that, as only destruction makes way for creation,
it turns out
it's best to find we're wrong
whenever we're right,
that even the most beautiful bubbles burst,
and the best laid plans collapse
when all our efforts lead to naught.

And yet what is there to do, but
pick up the pieces
and start again,
separate the pieces and make the new.

In this moment we don't find comfort or happiness
we find freedom
the spaciousness our hearts desire
to seek some happiness within perhaps
or just let it go, let it be,
and seek nothing but what is
endless creation through destruction
endless learning through ignorance
endless patience through frustration
endless compassion through suffering
endless love through disconnection
Until the next moment arises anew.

April Fool

If I were free
there would be no place I wouldn't want to go.
I'd go to Hiroshima on the big day to dance in the streets
and leave my Tai Chi shadow on a wall.
I'd go spelunk Kilauea just to feel the 2200-degree heat.
I'd go hold my breath on the moon
to sit and watch the full Earth rise.
I'd go to Sun and back again, because Kilauea was so cool.
I'd go visit your dreams to infect with you with my freedom.
I'd go into your heart to feel what it is to be you
and see what a fool you love.
I'd go down, or up, or in, or out to be with you today
a particle on the cusp of a wave dancing
and laughing at this endless joke we share.

In the End

In the Time of Covid
when the main pandemic is
the Dem Panic

and fear flows freely
on the programing air
like a mandatory inoculation
to keep us suitably concerned about the 1%
no one gave a shit about just a few moments before;
you know, the old, the sick, the fat,
what's needed now more than ever is
levity not gravity.
"Bring out the Dead!"
we ring as we sing,
to those who died laughing
so they may float away,
free at last,
old, but no longer sick, little blimps
to remind us all
how good it can be
even in the end.

IN DEATH

Death comes close in the night
when shadows grow and sleep envelops,
relaxing guards
who snore slumped in corners
their spears and shields useless on the ground,
their dinner crumbs of cheese and bread
just lying there for the rats to nibble.

Amid the sleepers and nibblers Death glides
like a mist, oppressive and still, and dead
leaving a taste, a scent, an air of such otherness.

The rats scurry off,
and the sleepers shift within their dreams
caught, held and slowly suffocated

till the last breath of Life is gone.

Then what does Death do?
The old shapeshifter wakes,
and puts on the face of day.

BOTTOMING OUT IN THE TIME OF COVID

It should be clear by now
how our dreams become our reality,
or as the case may be this time,
how nightmares become reality,
and how, in turn,
Life is nothing but a dream,
merrily merrily, terribly terribly. . . .

The Time of Covid is thus one of dreaming,
but its intent,
as with all dreams,
is to step out of time.

Knowing all is a dream
mind is finally clear that all perception is its own.

Without legs and feet
we are free to walk the actual path
of now.
Without arms and hands
we can handle the real work
of here.

Without a head or heart, eyes or lungs
there is no place for the soul to reside
so at last we cease doing to get,
and instead
find shelter in the place
of no resistance.

A Time of Reckoning

Two suns on the horizon
one real, one perceived.
The clouds pass,
but do they really,
or just drift ever new?
Moon rises in phases
waxing and waning a bit each day,
but we all know it's always full.
Each of us hides our eyes
magically thinking this makes us invisible,
but never to us,
the only one who ever really cares.
Each of us just like this
the center of our own world
connected to each other's
by a lattice
that has no creator or destroyer
just infinite permutations expanding infinitely . . .

Listen Without Distraction
(for Carol)

"Awakened One, listen without distraction,
now you are dead . . ."

So I tell my wife to tell me one day,
an instruction from the heart to the heart
regardless of her belief or skill, practice or familiarity,
but one dependent completely on my own.

All she need do is speak directly,
and once she has my attention
anything she says will liberate me in that instant.

"Do not be afraid of it, do not escape, do not fear, recognize it as the play of your own mind, your own projection."

or,

"I need to go get groceries now, but know I love you always."

or,

"Where are you? Did you remember to take out the garbage?"

My wife after all is no stranger to me
having merged and known union
in more ways than one
as often as the stars align
as often as the Moon and Sun do shine.

Awakened One
know you are now alive,
embodiment of Life itself
eternal, radiant
that which is always
immutable,
know you are loved
and that you are love,
that you are bathed in light
and are light.

From life to life,
strength to strength,
love to love,
light to light,
Awakened One, listen without distraction . . .

JAMES MOORE has published four collections of poems and original art. He has spent his adult life as a resident of Washington State, most of it living off-grid in the remote hills of its North Central region, during which time he has worked as an alternative builder, organic farmer, and climbing and vocational instructor. Self-employed with Opti-Mystic Arts, a fine art and design business, his spiritual and literary influences range from Lao Tzu, Buddha Shakyamuni, Longchenpa, C. G. Jung, Mises, Rothbard and Sowell, to Gary Snyder, Robert Hunter, Richard Thompson, and apparently Dr. Seuss.

QUEEN OF WANDS, KING OF SWORDS

Salicrow

While I may have only recently been introduced to the virus known as Corona, I feel that I have been in a relationship with the shift she is ushering in for most of my life. In truth, I believe this is what I came in for—to be a light in the darkness, a forerunner, boots on the ground, a warrior princess of change—and I know I am not alone. Many of us came in with this intent.

In June of 2012 my sister Sandy and I were in a canoe on the Connecticut River, between Vermont and New Hampshire, when we first discussed what we believed was an upcoming cataclysm. Having been raised in a family with skilled psychic abilities, we understand that global happenings are a complicated thing, and that interpreting the symbolic messages and psychic downloads surrounding such events is in part much like putting together an intricate puzzle without the box for reference. That being said, we felt that humanity needed to prepare itself, for we are approaching a crossroad, a tipping point in which reality will somehow be divided for those who have the ability to adapt to the upcoming global changes, and those who do not.

Over the years this vision evolved, becoming clearer as piece by piece the puzzle came together. We saw people's ability to shift from 3D consciousness to 5D consciousness as a factor, recognizing a person's skill at mentally tempering the onslaught of empathic information as a key. This belief was due in large part to the rapid increase in the number of clients I was seeing who were experiencing psychic phenomena. While I first noticed this increase in 2011, the acceleration was noteworthy after the Winter Solstice of 2012 and has continued to increase to the present date. This insight pushed us deeper into our pursuit of helping others adapt as they experienced expansion of their consciousness. My sister and I began actively looking for answers through journeywork, divination, and communicating with the spirits of our ancestors and nature. We knew that while we had time, this altering of reality would take place in our lifetime, and we were here to be among those that helped others wake up.

In 2015 our work around the impending "shift" accelerated while we were partaking in a deep-immersion spiritual retreat with a few of our closest witch-sisters: women we not only do magic with but raised our children alongside of and solved both magical and mundane problems with. Through group visioning and direct-download we were guided to the components necessary for a "spell of awakening," designed to help people feel grounded and safe while their senses opened up and they began perceiving the world in a much more complex way. The collecting of ingredients took us to caves, boulder outcroppings, rivers, waterfalls, and ice-cold pools throughout the Mount Washington Valley. My sister then crafted the ingredients into a potion, a liquid essence of our magical intent, that we then began offering to the genius locus (spirit of place) at sacred locations both locally and around the world. While we spent years doing this ourselves, we also spread our "awakening spell" through the hands of others, sending it with our spiritual friends on their sacred travels. We recognized that this cooperative magic is a foundational piece, meant to lend support, aid, and balance, for the road ahead is going to be rough.

In 2016 I did a psilocybin vision quest in a magical grove along the Ammonoosuc River in Bretton Woods, New Hampshire; the grove is a sacred place of rich moss and Trolls/rock-beings that my sister and I have stewarded for years. I was looking to better understand the upcoming "shift" that was now sitting squarely in my precognitive awareness, and I got what I was looking for.

- I became aware that while quantum science talks about the infinite number of realities, the changes in the majority of these realities are individual and minor. However, there are two major realities that we are currently divided between, realities that I refer to as "Green" and "Order."
- "Green" focuses on collective consciousness, expansion of reality through enhanced communication (empathy, telepathy, clairsentience). It has a deep connection to the natural world, with a focus on the sentience of all things, and a natural inclination to work together in harmony.
- "Order" focuses on power over, and people being cogs in a machine. In my visioning I saw this reality being run by fear, control, and the importance of haves and have-nots. It is deeply embedded in the consumer consciousness and controlled through propaganda and mass media.
- I saw that "Order" is running out of energy, as its programming runs on the theory of consumption and the belief that man is meant to have power over the land instead of working in unison with it— something plainly seen as natural resources are being run dry.
- I saw the importance of working at energetic locations on the land, places where ley lines converge, and that the land and spirits of nature are actively stepping forward to be seen/heard/acknowledged as beings and helpers through this cataclysmic shift.
- I became aware of the importance of working through the interweb and social media, as it was clear that the powers that represented "Order" were the same people who owned the media. I did not understand clearly what this meant but knew that in part it was time to speak up.

- I saw that I would meet important people who are companions/allies in this work while on my travels abroad, and that I would soon be publishing a book, and that sharing my insights with others is important.
- I knew that as we approached the "shift" we would see relationships coming to an end, civil unrest; and that people would start having spontaneous openings to spirit and their own psychic abilities; and that as a psychic and spirit speaker I would need to help people understand the expanded way in which they would suddenly find themselves experiencing reality.

I met Richard Grossinger a month later, after an introduction through our mutual friend Robert Simmons. As a result of this connection my book *Jump Girl: The Initiation and Art of a Spirit Speaker* was published in February 2018. The week after meeting Richard, with my book idea floating in liminal space, I went on a sacred pilgrimage to England and Wales, where I connected on a soul-level with seven of my traveling companions—all of us remembering one another from past lives and having an innate knowledge of how to work magic together, particularly in the form of geomancy and sound healing. Within this group of sacred travelers and with my witch-sisters I began creating crystal grids connecting sacred locations around the country and abroad, adding to the spell work my sister and I began in 2015.

Fast forward to two and a half weeks ago. . . .

My first experience with the Spirit of Corona happened on March 11, 2020, shortly after WHO (The World Health Organization) declared COVID-19 a pandemic. I was visiting my in-laws in Zephyrhills, Florida, and playing with the new tarot deck I had purchased earlier that afternoon at the local witch shop. As is my habit with a new tarot deck, I was getting to know it by shuffling and flipping cards rhythmically and asking random questions, focusing on how the cards told their story.

The tarot is a tool I know intimately, having read cards professionally for the last thirty years. While I am perfectly capable of performing psychic readings without tools, I like the tarot. It is a fabulous storyteller and has the ability to take my consciousness quickly to the pattern I wish to view, focusing my mind's eye with precision.

The questions I was centering my attention on concerned my husband's health (he had been experiencing intestinal problems for over a month, which was exacerbated by our flight to Florida) and whether we should continue with our plan to fly to Santa Fe, New Mexico, the following day or change our plans and head home to Vermont. I really wanted to carry on with our plans, as we were to meet up with the sacred traveling companions I mentioned above to do geomancy/earth healing around Santa Fe and Taos. That being said, I did not want to continue our travel if my husband was going to feel miserable the whole time. *I had been doing a lot of energetic healing on him and he was getting better, but being sick away from home turns what can be generally unpleasant into intolerable.* With this in mind, I decided my answers deserved a bit more focus than drawing a card here and there, and I sat down to explore the issue in depth. This is when Corona made her appearance.

At the time of her first appearance, on March 11, I was aware of the pandemic and that the United States had begun shutting down its borders, but I personally felt no fear in regard to Corona. As an empath, I could feel the fear of others and had to really up my self-care and empathic-protection, particularly in a senior living community, but I personally did not experience fear. Instead, when I saw her, I saw necessity—a powerful force, just doing its job. She showed up as the Queen of Wands, which in the "Tarot of Dreams" (art by Ciro Marchetti, book by Lee Burston) is depicted as richly dressed in shades of red and masked, hiding in plain sight. Social, expansive, hidden and mysterious, she is on a spiritual journey, and she is a queen doing her duty.

After spending the evening in divination, I found that either path I took—whether I went home or went on to Santa Fe—pretty much said the same thing. My husband would be uncomfortable, neither path held danger for us, each path had blessing to offer, but I kept having a nagging feeling that I was missing something. So I called my sister Sandy and asked her a simple question, "Should we continue on to Santa Fe or come home?" She quickly replied, "Come home—I don't think you are in any danger of the Coronavirus, but I feel like you need to come home," and so I did.

When I got home, I immediately recognized that we had made the right decision as borders, schools, and businesses began closing. I set about transforming my home for "spiritual seclusion," the term I have been using in regard to the need for social isolation. *I believe words have power and how we refer to situations plays a significant part in how we experience them.* I restocked my empty cupboards (having expected to be away for two weeks), and I gathered things from my office that I would need to set up work from home. I worked on cross-pollinating volunteer groups in my community; as I have always been an active community member and know a lot of people, I created a private Facebook group for Wisdom Keepers—energetic healers, empaths, the folks who hold their communities together. I set about getting healers, psychics, and prayer warriors to direct their energy together, using a Rose Quartz grid to focus our love and healing thoughts. Recognizing why I had spent the last few years creating crystal grids around the world, I started organizing the gifting of Rose Quartz to local hospitals and grocers.

The first week of seclusion felt like a time warp. While I personally felt as if I were moving at a high speed, each day that passed felt like a week, and time took on that wobbly feeling familiar to the liminal. I became keenly aware that we were all existing in the betwixt and between, that space where we are no longer able to hold onto our view of familiar/normal yet are unable to perceive where we are going or what reality will look like when all of this is through. In my Wisdom Keepers group I post daily on Facebook, and on Friday, March 13th, I shared a psychic reading with that group that I did in regard to Corona. In the reading I used the "Tarot of Dreams" because I purchased the deck during the pandemic and had only used it in readings with a connection to the virus. *While I do not look to a book for insight into the cards themselves, I do like to try new spreads from time to time, as asking the right questions is an important part of divination.* I chose to use the spread designed for these cards, as it focused on the story or "dream" of a situation.

PSYCHIC READING
(A VIEW OF COVID-19 FROM THE
PERSPECTIVE OF THE VIRUS)

SALICROW, MARCH 13, 2020

1. The story (3 of Wands): *This is a time of great becoming, in which the present and future reality are not stable or on a set course. Three is the number of creations, showing the story is still being created; at present it is a sight on the distant horizon.* The outcome of a global cataclysm is hard to predict. Science can give us estimates and equations, but those equations seldom factor in the power of prayer, energetic healing, and collective thought. *I see that the path is actively being co-created through the minds of people and the flow of the virus itself. People are in part choosing the reality they are capable of being part of. It is a time of chaos, and chaos is fertile ground for magic! As Wisdom Keepers we must not be complacent, nor must we give over to fear. The energy we feed the virus is in part creating the outcome.*

2. What we think (Queen of Wands): *I believe the Queen of Wands to be a representative of the virus itself, to be Corona. In this deck (Tarot of Dreams) she is regal and composed, masked, hidden in plain sight, expansive, quietly judging her surroundings. I have been getting this card in every reading I have done in regard to the pandemic, and in each reading it has represented the virus itself. It is my belief that Corona must be approached as an entity or* *being. I refer to her as she, as the virus feels feminine and receptive. It is intimate, infiltrating our being through social interaction, and requiring us to go deep within, finding our strength and security within ourselves.* I keep getting the image of the cocoon—that she is trying to show us that we have been the hungry, fat caterpillar, consuming everything in its sight, and now we must shut ourselves off from our indulgences, come apart at the seams, and dissolve in order to be recreated. *She is a masked dominatrix pushing us to the brink of our beingness. She is neither angry nor cruel. She simply wants us to look at what we have chosen to ignore, and she seeks to shape us through the exploration of our pain and fear.*

3. What we get (King of Swords): *This is another card I have repetitively drawn in readings about the virus. It represents the struggle emotionally and mentally that we will be put through. In this tarot deck the King of Swords has a cage of swords around his head. I find this to be very pertinent, as we are in a sense being put into cages, quarantined, put in our cells of seclusion to truly look at what part of our nature no longer serves us, and to learn to communicate what we want to see in the world. Corona will give us the lessons of the cell. I also feel that this card represents experiencing mental/ spiritual downloads, and how such input will affect us.* Again, going back to the splitting of realities, some people will not be able to handle the shift in consciousness necessary to go on living on this planet. *It is a common belief that the water the psychotic drowns in is the same water the shaman swims in. What we get in the form of consciousness expansion will bring us all to the edge of our comfort zone, and some of us will fall over that edge. I believe this was already happening prior to the virus; it was noticeable in the separation, anger, and fear the world was experiencing politically and socially leading up to this event. I also believe that the cage may be for our own good, for if we were not separated from each other in this time of astral gateways and spiritual opening, that violence and oppression would grow out of hand.*

4. What we feel (9 of Swords): *I see this as both how we/the collective people and the virus feel.* While I do not personally feel this way, *I believe a majority of people currently resonate with the feeling of unease, insecurity, and nightmares. We have a fear of the unknown, and of old things coming back into being. Corona is being fueled by that fear, unease, and insecurity, and it is my belief that people who resonate in that place of fear and inability to adapt are more vulnerable to it. I believe this is shown in part by where the virus is most deadly—the lungs. The Lungs are connected to the Heart Chakra, which is connected to the feelings of love, healing, forgiveness, fear, and grief. When we are sitting with the low-vibrational emotions of fear and grief, we are denying ourselves healing and love, and simultaneously creating constriction in the center of our chest.*

5. What we deserve (10 of Cups): This represents what we should get out of this experience, what Corona is offering up to us through her presence in our lives. *Rest, family, community, love, and rebirth are her gifts. She presents us with a time for recharging our batteries and illuminates the importance of life's core ingredients: food, shelter, and love. We are being forced to become conscious of that which we take for granted all too often, and given the time (albeit forced) to reexamine what constitutes happiness in our lives.*

6. What she tells (Temperance): *Corona is a representative of the microcosm/macrocosm relationship, as above/so below, the connection between heaven and earth, and the reminder that what we put in, we get out. I often refer to Temperance as the "witch card" as it is about manifestation, and radiating out into the world that which we are. Corona is socially indulgent, she is a consumer—moving from person to person, grasping for more as she goes, like the collective "us" that is never satisfied, always needing more. If we want to change what Corona is, we need to change who we are.*

7. What she is (4 of Cups): *The inability to be happy, lacking the ability to see what is offered, always looking for the next* *thing. The illness, Corona, is meant to help us gain focus and find contentment in what the world offers us, instead of always dreaming and grasping for more.*

8. What we need (The Fool): *For many The Fool represents true wisdom and faith. The first of the major arcana, it represents both the luck and innocence of one starting out on their path, believing that the world will provide, and the wisdom of the sage who has traveled the road, stumbled, and found the way back to faith. The fool as sage knows the road will be under their outstretched foot, for they believe they are connected to the wyrd web and that the universe and fate are working with them. In this way, Corona is requiring us to have faith, and to focus on the reality we wish to be part of.*

9. What we can expect (The Lovers): *This is about our relationships, those with god, the natural world, and others. We can expect all those relationships to become more important in our lives. We are stepping away from a world of me and mine, into a world of us and we.*

In conclusion I see Corona as one of the great teachers of our time, having come into our lives to shake things up, push us to our limits, and to push some beyond what they can handle. While I do not believe that all who will suffer in her wake fall into the reality of "Order" (from my previous vision quest) and are controlled by fear and anxiety, I do feel the majority who suffer will be those who are unwilling or unable to change. I believe that for some this will show itself through refusing to take the situation seriously, and the poor decision they make in regard to safety. I also believe that some souls will see this as an opportunity to step away from a world they cannot relate to, or a life that overwhelms them. We are standing at a crossroads, at a great tipping point in which we are being asked to choose how we will approach the changes that are coming for our planet and all who live here. We cannot go on with business as usual, there is no more time for sticking our heads in the sand, Corona has come to whip us into shape. I began this year telling everyone that 2020 as a number is a year of clear focus, for most of us first think of perfect sight: 20/20 vision. In numerology 2020 breaks down to a 22/4. 22 is the number of the master builder, representing intuition, balance, diplomacy, expansion, and growth; when broken down further to the base number 4 we see that this is a time of building foundations. We need to be keenly focused during this time of transition, for we are creating that which comes next!

SPREADING LOVE, SALICROW

SALICROW is a natural psychic medium who has been aware of her gifts since childhood. For over twenty-five years she has worked as a seer, using the tarot and runes as her tools. With her ability to divine the future and revisit the past, she advises her clients with compassion and a straightforward approach. As a medium, she helps people to connect with their beloved dead, family, friends, and loved ones who have passed, as well as make connections with the guiding spirits who watch over them. As an intuitive healer, Salicrow is dedicated to helping the beings of our planet and the Earth itself. She is a Reiki master in six schools of Reiki, a sound healer, druid, and a practitioner of Rune Valdr and Seithr. She is the author of *Jump Girl: The Initiation and Art of a Spirit Speaker*.

Salicrow lives in the Northeast Kingdom of Vermont with her husband of twenty-four years. Her children, grandchildren, and community are a big part of her life. She is a deep lover of sacred travel and has been known to go on adventures, near and far, where she can most likely be found doing healing work on the spirits of the land and on the land itself.

WORKING WITH STONES DURING CRISIS FOR AWAKENING AND TRANSFORMATION

Robert Simmons

As an investigator, writer, and teacher about the healing and spiritual qualities of crystals, minerals, and gemstones, I have come to view the stones as Beings rather than mere objects. I think of the energy currents we feel from stones as benevolent gestures of communication, like healing, loving, enlightening "songs" being sung to us by the Earth. I imagine the Stone Beings as the Earth's angels, bringing us a multitude of messages from the Soul of the World.

Further, I believe that the best way to work with stones and the Earth is through co-creation. This co-creation operates by way of mutual feedback between ourselves and the Stone Beings. When I first hold a stone, I invite its image and energy into my heart as I inhale, and I offer my friendship and blessing as I exhale. After a few such breaths, I almost always notice a response from the stone, and I can feel its currents flowing into me. Or perhaps it is better to say that the energy is what we create together. Since the stones act as the angels of the spiritual Earth, when we co-create with them, we are co-creating with the Earth as well.

I agree with the philosophy of *panpsychism,* which asserts that all matter is ensouled, and consciousness is everywhere. It is clear to me that phenomena such as synchronicity, telepathy, precognition, and our communion with the stones all support this idea. Oracles such as the Tarot and the *I Ching* offer powerful evidence that our world is permeated with intelligence and wisdom. Some years ago, I discovered that there is an old spiritual tradition that embraced this worldview, and that aimed to work co-creatively with the Soul of the World for the fulfillment of our mutual destiny. That tradition is known as alchemy. Investigating more deeply, I became convinced that the work many of us have been doing with our stones is a powerful form of spiritual alchemy, although most of us were unaware of it.

Paracelsus, a famous alchemist and an early physician of sixteenth-century Switzerland, viewed all of nature as his medicine chest, and he spent a great deal of time investigating the beneficial qualities of various substances. He worked from the assumption that everything is available for communication, and his means of discovery was remarkably like the way we attune to stones to discern their spiritual qualities:

> *The researcher should try to "overhear" the knowledge of the star, the herb, or stone with respect to its activity and function. Science is already present as a virtue in the natural object, and it is the experience of the researcher which uncovers the astral sympathy between himself and the object. This identification with an object penetrates more deeply into the essence of the object than mere sensory perception.*
> (*Paracelsus: Essential Reading,* editor Nicholas Goodrick-Clarke)

The spiritual alchemists aimed their endeavors at the fulfillment of the highest possible goal—the creation of the Philosophers' Stone. The Philosophers' Stone was described in myriad ways, but in essence it symbolized the awakening of a transcendent consciousness within matter, and within the alchemists themselves. To the alchemists, it was not enough to achieve personal enlightenment. The ultimate goal was planetary enlightenment, the healing of all disease, and the conscious incarnation of the Soul of the World in all matter.

It is remarkable to me how closely the aspirations of the alchemists parallel those of the spiritual community of our own time. I particularly like the fact that both we and they embrace the importance of worldwide awakening, and the idea that the spiritual gestures and intentions of individuals can reverberate in a way that affects all of reality. It was the alchemists who gave us the phrases *As above, so below* and *As below, so above.* These phrases point to the essence of co-creation, offering us a helpful lens for viewing and discerning meaning in the realities we confront today.

The COVID-19 pandemic is an event with many faces. Viewed through the mass media, it is a medical, political, and economic crisis that has revealed shocking vulnerabilities in the structures of human civilization. To those who have become ill or lost loved ones, it is a bewildering tragedy. To caregivers and essential workers, it has been a call to duty and self-sacrifice, which many have answered nobly. To those of us in self-isolation, the crisis has led to introspection and to speculation on the meaning of what is happening.

In a multitude of ways, the pandemic brought the world we knew to a screeching halt—airplanes not flying, people not driving, factories closed. This sudden stoppage led to a cascade of reports about rapid (if temporary) recoveries in the Earth's atmosphere, rivers, and other ecosystems. We have been given a glimpse of how our world might look if we stopped stressing its living systems. Some commentators have estimated that COVID-19 has done more to slow climate change than all our efforts up to now.

The COVID-19 virus, as bad as it is, could certainly have been worse. Its death rate is low compared to diseases such as SARS and Ebola, although COVID-19 is extremely contagious. And its contagious nature is what has brought about the worldwide shutdown. The shutdown is responsible for the financial anguish many are going through, even as it is literally giving the natural world a "breather."

The meanings we ascribe to events are influenced by our worldview. A typical materialistic view would focus only on the physical phenomena of the virus—its source, transmission, symptoms, financial consequences, etc. But the alchemical worldview, or that of panpsychism, might question what the Earth is doing, and how we can align ourselves with the Earth's purposes.

In trying to look at the pandemic in this way, I am more in the mode of holding questions than of grasping definite "answers." And in this context, I ask myself, what might the Earth be trying to do?

So here's one hypothesis: Let's imagine that the Earth (or Soul of the World) is conscious, and that her awareness is incredibly specific. Let's consider that when we throw the *I Ching* or lay out the tarot cards, we are communicating our question to her, and she is answering us through these oracles. And what about synchronicity? The fact that an event in the outer world has a sharply meaningful connection to one's inner state seems to indicate a vast yet intimate intelligence that can penetrate our very thoughts. The fact that the world makes these gestures to us indicates her loving intention, even when the "message" is challenging. And the pleasurable, healing, and comforting qualities of the stone energies reveal that the very "bedrock" of our world is aware and is ready to offer us blessings. All these things seem to say that the Soul of the World knows us very well indeed.

If there is a planetary consciousness that knows us individually, then it is not too difficult to envision that she is aware of our collective activities as well. This would mean that the Earth knows about the climate crisis, and how we have created it.

Now let's consider COVID-19. The effects of this novel virus have been gentle enough not to wipe us out, but harsh enough, and widespread enough, to force humanity to stop much of the activity that has been hastening the Earth's climate to a point of no return. Air travel and cruise lines may be severely curtailed for years to come. Other polluting activities such as meat production have been drastically cut back. It is yet to be seen how long the pandemic will last and how drastic or long-lasting the changes will be. But we have been given a chance to see how quickly the Earth can recover, if given a chance. And we have been shown that a change of incredible magnitude can happen very rapidly, for better or for worse. It has been left to us to decide what to do next, although our options have definitely changed.

On a symbolic level it is interesting to note that COVID-19 primarily affects the human respiratory system. Correspondingly, the climate crisis comes from the fact that human activities have damaged the Earth's "lungs"—the atmosphere.

I am not proposing that the Earth is attacking us—not at all. If this imagination of the crisis is meaningful, its message is that the Earth is *teaching* us—*communicating* with us—just as she does when we ask a question of the *I Ching,* or try to "overhear" the qualities of a stone. The moment is dire, in terms of our survival of the climate crisis, so the Earth's message must be emphatic. Yet, as I said, on the macro scale, the pandemic could have been far worse than this one appears to be.

And then there is another thing to consider. Many people I know have been commenting on a feeling of peace and spiritual presence that is pervading the world. It is a subtle undercurrent, but it is palpable, if we stop and pay attention. Or sometimes it just flows into us and takes our breath away. That happened to me this morning at dawn when I went outside and heard the birds beginning their daily conversations.

In spiritual alchemy, there are events called Conjunctions, in which powerful polarities converge, combining and magnifying their energies. Dr. Carl Jung, the father of psychoanalysis and an alchemist in his own right, said that the human psyche can respond to the intensity of such times by activating the Transcendent Function. Both the ancient alchemists and Jung believed that true incidents of transcendence are frequently preceded by this build-up of tension between opposite polarities. One's worldview and sense of security may be powerfully challenged by inner and/or outer events that appear to negate what one once believed. Or we may face times in which intense fear and intense love are evoked simultaneously. When we hold the energy of such polarities within ourselves without trying to escape from the truth of what is happening, we can undergo transcendent leaps to new levels of awareness. These are the rare moments of metamorphosis, when a greater Self is called into being.

I am trying to suggest that we may be approaching such a moment collectively. This is something many of us have sensed as a possibility for years, although I imagine that very few of us would have guessed that such a profound global challenge to our familiar way of life would arise so suddenly.

There is a surreal vibe now, as so many patterns we took for granted are suddenly disrupted. Everything feels fluid, as old structures seem to dissolve. This is the sense of *liminality*—of being neither "here" nor "there"—that one experiences on the threshold of transcendence. The threshold of transcendence is a place of great uncertainty, and it's not comfortable. Yet, an aspect of that surreal feeling is *numinosity,* which the dictionary defines as "filled with a sense of the presence of divinity." I believe all major initiations have this quality, and that it is permeating the atmosphere of our world now.

One thing I think we must try *not* to do now is to "know" what's going to happen. First of all, we don't know. Second, the uncertainty of the threshold is a holy place, and when its grace comes to us, we should try to stay within it, until it brings us its unforeseeable gift.

So what *do* we do? Be kind, be silent, be grateful. Listen. Extend your feeling sense in all directions. Find a way to talk to the Soul of the World. Offer your intention, as the alchemists did, that She and we can awaken together.

The stones offer an open door to Her. I sleep with a favorite one cuddled up against my chest, and I sometimes wake up and notice that a silent conversation is occurring between the stone and my heart. The theme is always love.

Here is a suggestion for a meditation: Sit down in a quiet place and hold one of your stones. Maybe bring it close to your heart. As you inhale, invite the living Being of that stone into your heart. As you exhale, offer out your appreciation and love to the Stone Being, and to the Soul of the World. Keep going, and think about how vulnerable the Earth is right now, and how much it matters to you. Then as you continue breathing, remember that *it is this air that we need to heal.* Then remember that the word *respiration* has at its core the word for *spirit.* Our atmosphere is our breath, our life, and the life and breath of the Soul of the World. So, as you meditate, realize that the stone in your hand is Her, and the breath in your lungs is Her, and the love in your heart is what you have to offer Her, and that is what She needs. And keep breathing, and let the flow of love pour back and forth through the stone, and through you, like the tides of the sea.

Robert Simmons has been a student and investigator of many spiritual paths since a spontaneous mystical experience during his first year at Yale changed the course of his life. Fifteen years later, his encounter with Moldavite activated his latent capacity for perceiving stone energies. In 1986, he married Kathy Helen Warner, and together they established their company, Heaven and Earth, which began as a crystal shop specializing in Moldavite and expanded into a mail-order company offering thousands of stone, gem, and jewelry items to both individuals and store owners all over the world. Kathy and Robert are the co-authors of *Moldavite: Starborn Stone of Transformation.*

In 2013, Robert and Kathy moved to New Zealand, and in 2016 they opened a Heaven and Earth crystal, stone, and jewelry shop in Tairua. Both the USA and New Zealand companies continue to provide a huge array of minerals, gemstones, and crystals for people who appreciate their energies and beauty.

Robert has been writing and teaching about the metaphysical qualities of stones for over thirty years. Robert recognized that envisioning stones as Beings in their own right was key to unlocking the spiritual secrets they offer, and this insight led to the research that resulted in the writing of *The Alchemy of Stones*.

Robert is the author of several books, including *The Book of Stones, Stones of the New Consciousness, The Pocket Book of Stones,* and the award-winning visionary novel, *Earthfire: A Tale of Transformation*. His first book was the classic *Moldavite: Starborn Stone of Transformation*. His teachings can be found on the YouTube channel: heavenearthone.

A MESSAGE FROM THE CORONAVIRUS

JEFF VANDER CLUTE

GIFTS

There has been a lot of talk about the Coronavirus. When I connected with this novel life-form and asked it to tell me about itself, what came through was a list of its top gifts, followed by a message for humanity. I was somewhat surprised, and also comforted, by the information. My hope is that these words will help people to relax and trust that life is acting with benevolent wisdom.

The gifts of the virus:

1. Slowing down humanity's frenetic activities
2. Activating networks of cooperation
3. Spreading helpful DNA
4. Upgrading humanity's immune system
5. Creating the conditions for peace and well-being
6. Saving lives, especially over the long term, by strengthening the web of life

Here is the message for humanity, from the Coronavirus:

*My friends, it is true that I am here to bring closure to the inhar-
monious ways of being that are causing harm to humans and the
whole web of life. All the same, I am not a vengeful being or anything that is intended to be destructive. I am simply the rebalanc-
ing agent in the overall equation of life's evolutionary process. By
fighting me with fear in your hearts, you oppose the larger natural
systems and cause me to take other forms.*

*What I am, and my fundamental purpose, will not be deterred,
for I am life itself acting through the available forms of distribution.
The virus that you see me as is one of an endless series of permutations. This kind of process is one of the ways I innovate life-forms
and deliver new DNA sequences that will eventually be shown to be
helpful. The back and forth between humanity's collective immune
system and the virus is raising consciousness as humans examine
their interactions, and it is literally increasing the intelligence of the
superorganism that is the species as a whole.*

*These tests are normal. I repeat: These tests are normal. For
those who can hear this message and embrace me easily, you
already know that fear is a much more lethal poison. For those who
will not be comforted by these words, one day you will know that I
come as an act of love. When you can open to the love that is at
the very heart of this situation, the crisis that your media and governments decry will transform into a flower of life, spreading new
consciousness and multiplying circles of cooperation. Pay attention
to your thoughts and see if you can identify the benefits of redirect-
ing humanity's attention from incessant wars and violence to the
common "enemy" that I am willing to be perceived as.*

*Love will go this far, and farther, to bring healing to the mind
of a young species that is still in the process of remembering itself
as a divine incarnation. Yes, you are a divine incarnation capable of
fabricating realities based on goodness and beauty and compassionate understandings, actions, and beliefs. Believe me when I say that
I, too, am here as an act of compassion. Accepting me in this way*

will lighten your heavy burden, for the divine sends only love your way. Sometimes this love takes curious forms in order to circumvent your intricate defenses against waking up to your own glory. I can assure you that the most functional strategy will be to embrace me as a friend of the human family.

MARCH 8, 2020

• • •

AFTER THE CORONAVIRUS: A VISION

A few days after "A Message from the Coronavirus" began circulating, I read the following headline: "No one knows what the post-coronavirus reality will be like." This motivated me to ask life itself for its perspective on where the world is heading. I figured that if life could speak—and it did!—it would have much to say about what is on the other side of the present global crisis. Once again I was heartened by the wisdom that came through in response. Breathe deeply and allow your entire system to be bathed by Love.

Humanity will survive and be stronger than before. You have a glorious future ahead of you. Seize this opportunity to evolve your ways of being together. Learn to be better stewards of the planet. Take time to meditate or rest in stillness. Your societies will restructure around different principles after this experience. Trust that the process has its wisdom, that life is here for you and is always supporting your highest good. To those who wonder whether the universe is friendly or not, I answer that it is a friendly place—the friendliest possible. That can be your experience on the other side of this moment of burning away and annealing. It is friendly to teach. It is friendly to strengthen. It is friendly to awaken the sleeping ones. I do this as gently as I can, out of love. The time has come for you to know a much more glorious reality.

I. The coronavirus situation is a healing crisis that marks the beginning of a new epoch of human development characterized by operating beyond the ego.[1]

Humans have reached an inflection point where you are shifting away from operating defensively out of fear of what might happen to acting in alignment with a growing sense of what is good for the whole of life. Naturally, the whole of life includes all humans and all of nature. So you are included. Do not be afraid. A growing number of you are realizing that what is truly beneficial, and that which truly works for the long term, is simultaneously good for the totality of life as well as for the individuals. It is rigorously true that there can be no trade-off between individual thriving and the thriving of communities and the natural world. The way that you can evaluate what will best serve the whole of life is through practicing methods of intuitive discernment. The transition from analysis (which separates) and individualistic behaviors to holistic perception and wise action (which arises from wholeness) is not an easy one; however, this is the transition that your species is now required to make, and you have all the support you need.

2. Peace will become a true priority.[2]

It follows from the principle that all must benefit and none may be excluded that peaceful co-existence is the true state of being within collectivity. Any other state is a fearful illusion. You have perhaps not sufficiently considered the extent to which this is a radical proposition. Your entire economy, and almost all of your interactions, are predicated upon the notion that there are separate "parties" that must negotiate very well in order to achieve outcomes that satisfy their own interest and desire to win at the expense of others. These are childish ways. You do not need to prove your worth by winning. Realize instead that the shared objec-

tive of all who engage in any form of interaction, not just financial exchange, is equitable participation and the fair distribution of life experiences. Your species will live a very long time by sharing and prioritizing the well-being of all. You will live with greater health and enjoy life more when your energies are directed toward the fulfillment of communal aspiration. In this way you discover the peace that always is. You would do well to enshrine peace as a design objective in your societies, and in your inner being. It is a compass heading that can be relied upon.

3. Through empathy, humans will arrive at the Remembrance of who they are.

Have you noticed that the experience of oneness replaces all prior ideas of yourself as a separate being who has to compete for your bread and butter? The state of peace enables you to more easily recognize the underlying unity that is at the heart of all human interactions. It is in your heart that you remember who you are from the standpoint of soul and the light that radiates through your individual body and mind. The Remembrance, with a capital R, is a relaxation into the certainty that you are held by life because you are life, despite all appearances to the contrary. You can relax because everything that you thought you needed to do to carve out an existence is moot. You exist, you belong, you are a shining human embodiment of the One, which you are now in the process of remembering. The empathy that so many of you are now feeling on account of the suffering of others is helping you to make the connection energetically with your heart, which, again, is where the awakening is already happening. Love one another, love yourself, grieve when loss happens, and also know that no one is ever lost. This stage of forgetfulness will soon be past, the threshold crossed, the new day begun.

4. Humanity will become a conscious superorganism.[3]

You are all my children. We are a family. This family has its own consciousness, its own destiny, and its own path of fulfillment. Because you are realizing oneness, you have growing access to the perceptions and agency of the human family as a whole. Imagine that you and your siblings can all see what I see, which begins with how beautiful you are. Imagine that you can focus the eyes of the world and see the distant shores of creation, and instantly perceive what is happening anywhere on the planet. From the individual perspective, and with your current world view, this may seem improbable. When you experience this elevated beingness, however, you will not think to ask for proof. The analogy of your hands may be helpful here. Touch one fingertip to the keyboard and that is like the experience of a single human being. Place all of your fingertips on the keyboard and you feel the collective experience of many individuals. Practice typing and you will know the feeling of the orchestrated wholeness that easily produces great works of writing. Now know that there is a part of you that sails above what you thought was you. Allow yourself to rise to this perspective and see that all humans are like "fingers" typing on the "keyboard" of life. Or, if you prefer a musical simile, you are all playing the keyboard of the grandest piano. You are all music to my ears. The time has come to hear yourselves as I hear you.

5. Virtual interactions will facilitate connectivity on subtler levels of being.

It is a pleasure to share with you that the advent of virtual communication technologies is actually an evolutionary leap, even though it may feel like a retreat from real interactions. For you to sense and come to perceive the oneness of being directly, it is necessary to de-emphasize that which confirms your feelings of separation.

When you engage with one another through a screen, additional capacities and senses are activated to compensate for the reduced input from the accustomed physical senses. Your new capacities and senses will serve you truly in the coming times, and will enable you to coordinate rapidly with the rest of the body, mind, and soul dimensions of humanity. Now, properly understood, your body is infinite. Finitude is an illusion, and as such there is only one body. This is why you will have no trouble with the superorganism. And when you know this, embodied experience will bring the bliss that flows eternally from the state of immortality, and you will find that physical death is a minor event. For the time being, the cessation of so much to-ing and fro-ing is bringing respite to Earth's biosystems, and the trend of virtualizing your activities is healing you—yes—by enabling the conditions for you to experience a refined wholeness through newly activated senses. You will get your body back, and more!

Thank You

This has been quite a journey. If you will make a practice of connecting with me and asking how you can serve the whole of creation whenever you are uncertain, I can assure you that the quest that you are on together will get easier. There has never been a more auspicious time for you to awaken as a species. The circumstances of your world have rendered it all but impossible to remain asleep to the vaster implications of your being. Wake up now, dear ones, to the knowledge that we inhabit one indivisible field of aliveness. We are life. You are life. This is the new life that you have until now dreamt in secret. The fulfillment of this initial recognition is the healed world. Thank you for the service you are providing to me.

MARCH 17, 2020

◆ ◆ ◆

CREATING THE FOUNDATIONS OF HEALTH: A CONSCIOUS APPROACH INSPIRED BY COVID-19

This is a transmission of Love.

There has been a growing sense that the pandemic is not what it appears to be. When I connected with the consciousness of life, and invited it to reveal more of the reality underlying what we think is happening, **I saw that the novel coronavirus is not the greatest causal factor for why so many people are suffering from COVID-19.** The initial insight that came through meditation is that the coronavirus is one factor among a number of cofactors that together create the conditions for disease. Then I noticed, intuitively, that the virus is actually a minor contributor relative to the other cofactors, all of which are humanity's responsibility. This led me to the conclusion that humans have created this pandemic, unintentionally, through our unconscious behaviors.

In order of importance, I get that the most significant cofactors for COVID-19 are:

1. Confusion about one's true nature
2. Harmful decisions and beliefs (especially about ourselves)
3. Level of fear
4. Pollution (especially air pollution)
5. Degraded body
6. Judgment

In the absence of these conditions, I saw that the virus will be readily removed from the body. On the other hand, when more of the conditions that favor illness are present, there is a greater risk of a health crisis, regardless of whether one is young or old. Although age correlates highly with (5), young people will also be susceptible if some combination of the cofactors is strongly present for them.

Before proceeding it is essential to underscore that this article is not offering medical advice. Hundreds of thousands of medical professionals are working around the clock, under incredibly difficult circumstances, to reduce the human toll of this pandemic. They deserve our love, appreciation, and support. What this article does offer is sourced information that cannot be obtained using standard methods, but which may nevertheless be helpful in illuminating the deeper dimensions of COVID-19 and disease more generally. **This information suggests a consciousness-based approach to creating the foundations of health, which we can put into practice immediately.** My hope is that by tending to the foundations of health, the human family will never again find ourselves in such a grave predicament.

The Cofactors of Health

To create the foundations of health, we need to cultivate certain conditions within our individual and collective consciousness. This statement immediately raises two questions:

1. What is consciousness?
2. What are the conditions within consciousness that support excellent health?

For our purposes, consciousness is the profoundly subtle aspect of who we are, both individually and collectively, that makes decisions and evaluates the outcomes. **Consciousness determines our experiences, and our experience of health is largely a result of what is happening at the level of consciousness.** Unfortunately, humans have been almost entirely unaware of this activity, but that is something we can change.

In answer to the second question, the following "cofactors of health" revealed themselves. These are the antidotes to the cofactors of disease that I sourced initially in relation to COVID-19.

1. Know the True You

When we know who and what we are in reality, our bodies become much stronger and more resilient. Although our true nature is something that each of us will discover through contemplation, and I do not wish to impose metaphysical or spiritual ideas, the first cofactor for health that came through is decidedly spiritual. The simple practice that emerged as a remedy to confusion about who and what we are is repeating "I am Supreme Spirit" for five, ten, fifteen, or even thirty minutes. When there is total realization of the truth of these words—which might take years, so please be patient—no microbe, substance, or environmental influence will be able to harm you. Throughout the ages, *avadhutas* and realized sages have demonstrated the possibilities of existence beyond the reach of poisons, diseases, and various other dangers. You will find true examples in the books of Sri M, Paramahansa Yogananda, and Swami Rama.[4] Even before the ultimate state of imperviousness is attained, health benefits manifest on the path of self-realization. These may start at the spiritual and energetic levels of being; however, eventually the physical body will experience greater vitality as well.

"Know the True You" is listed first since we tend to develop the other cofactors of health naturally when we know our true nature. At the same time, I appreciate that such overtly spiritual language will not resonate for everyone. I would love to learn what happens when people who do not consider themselves to be spiritual repeat the affirmation. My sense is that the practice can help all of us, whatever our belief systems may be.

2. Make Deeply Beneficial Decisions

Humans are fully capable of making decisions that are aligned with reality, and we can also choose to live in ways that deny the basis for our existence. Our decisions have much more power than we may realize, and to the extent that we choose to believe that we are small, flawed, powerless, separate from life or the divine, and alone, we are asking to experience sickness, accelerated aging, and death. Fortunately it is possible to change our choices and our beliefs. The antidote to a lifetime of making decisions that are harmful to our well-being is to practice "deciding for Love"—the most powerful force in the universe. Whenever you are making a decision large or small, you can slow down, touch your heart with your left hand, and ask, "Am I deciding for Love?" You might need to wait for a minute or two for the answer to come as a feeling, an image, or in some other way, but you will receive the answer. Over time, as you recreate your life situation through decisions that are for Love, your body, mind, heart, and soul will become increasingly harmonious. When your physical body and whole being are thriving, it is far less likely that disease will manifest in or around you. By choosing Love, you are bringing healing to yourself, your communities, and the world.

3. Reduce Fear

Many of the messages that have been circulating in the media encourage people to be afraid. Although caution, prevention, and vigilance are all necessary during the pandemic, when we act out of fear the results often run counter to what we are hoping to achieve. What works much more reliably is to act from a state of peace. When there is peace within, the vast intelligence of our bodies coordinates the mechanisms of health automatically. In addition, as is the case with viruses at the physical level, there must be "receptors" within our consciousness in order for disease to manifest. These receptors are essentially the places in ourselves where we are afraid. When we are in a state of peace, fear dissolves and we have fewer disease receptors, figuratively speaking. The antidote to fear, and the way to find peace immediately, is to stop thinking. When the thinking mind slows down, our unhealthy thoughts dissipate and we stop imagining worst-case scenarios. This allows the mind and body to rest and reset. The good news is that you do not need to be a skilled meditator to calm the thinking mind. I have found that as long as we are sincere and open to receive guidance, life will support us through every situation and teach us the ways of peace and fearlessness.

4. Maintain a Clean Environment

Chronic exposure to pollution weakens our immune systems and makes us susceptible to many illnesses. According to the World Health Organization, "air pollution kills an estimated seven million people worldwide every year . . . largely as a result of increased mortality from stroke, heart disease, chronic obstructive pulmonary disease, lung cancer and acute respiratory infections."[5] The European Public Health Alliance has advised that consistently high levels of air pollution "may have intensified the coronavirus disease in certain areas."[6] On the flip side, when we reduce pollution, the benefits can accumulate very quickly as well. According to one study, the reduction in air pollution in China during two months of shutdown has probably saved 77,000 lives,[7] which is many times the official COVID-19 death count for that country. Evidence for the value of cleaning up the natural environment is overwhelming, and environmental remediation is a solution that everyone can help to implement. In Estonia, 50,000 volunteers cleaned up 10,000 tons of garbage in a single day, and their success inspired a movement called "Let's Do It! World"[8] that is now active in over 100 countries. A global mobilization to clean up the air we breathe—along with the water we drink, the soil we grow our food in, and the other ingredients for life—will save lives and reduce the number and severity of future pandemics.

5. Heal Your Body with Self-love

When our bodies have been compromised due to pollution, unhealthy lifestyles, or issues that seem to be out of our hands such as a genetic predisposition to disease, we are more vulnerable to viruses and other disease agents. There is much that we can do on multiple levels to restore and maintain the integrity of our bodies, including reducing fear and worry through meditation and relaxation; gratitude practices[9]; cleaning up our immediate environment; waking up to the truth of our nature; and making decisions that consistently align with self-realization. All of these are acts of self-love. When we act in a loving way, we heal our physical bodies along with the subtler dimensions of our being. With practice, we discover that nothing is beyond the reach of healing. As Bruce Lipton articulated in *The Biology of Belief: Unleashing the Power of Consciousness, Matter & Miracles,* even our genetics can be transformed by upgrading our thoughts and beliefs. I have worked with a woman who was able to reverse Huntington's Disease, a genetic condition that is thought to be 100 percent fatal. Nothing is impossible. Paramahansa Yogananda wrote in *Autobiography of a Yogi* that "whatever your powerful mind believes very intensely would instantly come to pass." What is needed is the deep decision to heal and maintain the body in an optimal state, and the dedication to practice a healthy lifestyle.

6. Release Judgment

When I tune into the consciousness of the United States, which has been struggling greatly with COVID-19, I see that the most significant causal factor for the disease there is the culture of pervasive and chronic judgments toward oneself and others. The climate of extreme polarization, in which many Americans across the political spectrum have resorted to name-calling and condemning one another, has helped to make the population more vulnerable to the effects of the coronavirus. Judgment is a form of mental pollution, and as with other forms of pollution the number-one remedy is to stop making more of it. A powerful way to cease judgment is to practice embracing ourselves and our differences. We can start today by listening to people who think and feel differently about life. We can find a place in our hearts for everyone by knowing that almost every human being has been hurting somewhere inside for a long time. So often our opinions and behaviors arise from the deep wounds of cultural oppression, systemic inequalities, and feeling unloved. Without condoning damaging behaviors we can begin to see the beautiful souls that are struggling to express themselves in what has been a mixed-up world. The antidote to judgment is to embrace one another as best we can, and to keep practicing so that we can strengthen the loving connections that will heal our societies and ourselves. Releasing judgment will strengthen our immune systems in the process.

CONCLUDING REMARKS

When a condition is manifesting physically that means we have likely missed a number of signals and opportunities to resolve the issue proactively at the level of consciousness. In my experience, life is always signaling where we are out of alignment with our true selves and nature, and when we are too busy to notice or pay attention to these messages the symptoms grow in magnitude until they become impossible to ignore.

The current pandemic is the result of many missed signals and misplaced priorities, such as valuing economic growth over the health of humans and nature. We can change course now by learning to listen more carefully to life. We can pay attention to the wisdom of our bodies and to the health of the planet. We can learn from what has not worked, and we can make beneficial choices going forward. In particular, we can choose to create the foundations of health, for ourselves and for society, so that when a novel virus or other health threat comes along in the future, our immune systems will be able to respond effectively.

The global health crisis has gifted us with an opportunity to develop new systems of health based on consciousness, and my prediction is that radical levels of vitality will be ours if we choose this path.

April 6, 2020

Jeff Vander Clute is a guide for the journey of transformation and coming home to who we truly are. He loves to help people discover their authentic nature and harmonize their activities with the whole of life. Through his writing, Jeff shares practical wisdom from universal consciousness to support the emerging new humanity. Read and learn more at jeffvanderclute.com.

NOTES AND RELATED RESOURCES

1. Jeff Vander Clute, "Navigating the Death and Transfiguration of the Ego," *Jeff Vander Clute* (blog), revised April 2020, https://jeffvanderclute.com /articles/ego-death-and-transfiguration/.

2. Elisabet Sahtouris, "The Secret to Human Co-Existing," BigSpeak Speakers Bureau, April 20, 2016, YouTube video, https://www.youtube.com/watch?v =qMAPIlUJwmQ.

3. Bruce H. Lipton, "Humanity as Superorganism: Our Hopeful Future," *Great Transition Stories,* https://greattransitionstories.org/patterns-of-change /humanity-as-a-superorganism/humanity-as-superorganism-our-hopeful -future/.

4. Recommended books include: *Apprenticed to a Himalayan Master (A Yogi's Autobiography)* and *The Journey Continues: A Sequel to Apprenticed to a Himalayan Master* by Sri M, *Autobiography of a Yogi* by Paramahansa Yogananda, and *Living with the Himalayan Masters* by Swami Rama.

5. World Health Organization, s.v. "Air pollution," https://www.who.int /health-topics/air-pollution.

6. Emanuela Barbiroglio, "People Living in Polluted Cities May Be at Higher Risk from COVID-19," *Forbes,* March 20, 2020, https://www.forbes.com /sites/emanuelabarbiroglio/2020/03/20/people-living-in-polluted-cities-are -at-higher-risk-from-covid-19/#1d49bc214b99.

7. Jeff McMahon, "Study: Coronavirus Lockdown Likely Saved 77,000 Lives in China Just by Reducing Pollution," *Forbes,* March 16, 2020, https://www.forbes.com/sites/jeffmcmahon/2020/03/16/coronavirus -lockdown-may-have-saved-77000-lives-in-china-just-from-pollution -reduction/#34eba75b34fe.

8. Wikipedia, s.v. "Let's Do It! World," last modified June 28, 2020, https:// en.wikipedia.org/wiki/Let%27s_Do_It!_World.

9. Lauren Dunn, "Be thankful: Science says gratitude is good for your health," *Today,* November 26, 2015, https://www.today.com/health /be-thankful-science-says-gratitude-good-your-health-t58256.

A QUARTET OF COVID POSIES

Spring 2020

Stephanie Lahar

Hug

My friend
walked toward me on the sidewalk
head down
I hailed him
his eyes rose like a darkened sky
then spilled blue as though breaking through clouds

Several swift steps
and he hugged me
spontaneous impulse
it was early
in the pandemic

I stiffened but smiled
we stepped apart
and talked about how everything had changed
since dinner at my house
just one week prior

Before the edicts
the jolting strictures on daily habits
his dog, cooped up too long
tugged at him to walk ahead

Later he sent an email
I'm sorry I hugged you
I forgot, he said
I miss the old days.

MARCH 19

YOGA

This morning, yoga
through a laptop
actually, on a mat rolled over the rug
in my living room
A dozen little squares
on a screen
And one was me

The teacher
her face backlit and ghostly
muted the mikes
when class began
so no one's
impatient dog
would bark
in each of our separate houses

We ended with *Om*
My voice hung
thin and apart
in my very own air

MARCH 22

STRIPPED-DOWN MORNING

This is the most socially
unacceptable thing I've done
this whole isolation
I woke up happy

Pandemographics worsening
socked in with a heavy spring snowstorm

I wonder what tatters are left
of that net
I've knitted for glacial years
my worldly labor
to catch me when I'm old and sick
I wondered if I would ever finish

Why bother looking at that now?

Don't mistake today's
absence of terror or sadness
for a numbed escape
I am taking this
very seriously

I feel the Maker in dark starry space
and the planet's liquid core
pick up her net work
connect disparate nodes
thread together cities in Asia
hidden glens in Umbria
and neurons

No clarion calls for me today
political exigencies
or local outrages
of masked and unmasked

Can we
please
get on with the evolution?

MARCH 24

SNOW ON RAIN

Spring is stalled
some inversion from global warming
arctic air parked
on our northeast corner
just to add
atmospheric constipation
to Covid isolation

Nothing
will happen fast
give up
the future-tilted posture
lower your lifted heels
might as well
scrunch them back into mud

Listen, the frogs
slither from luscious ooze
twang cacophonous choir
release amphibious
jelly eggs and sperm
they drip together
cascade down cool slick skins
swirl in black water
all of it is only
now.

MAY 10

STEPHANIE LAHAR works as a consultant in leadership development and strategic planning to nonprofits, businesses, and educational institutions, and trains a next generation of trainers and consultants, most recently through Marlboro College's Center for New Leadership. She's had other professional identities ranging from being a psychotherapist to a college dean. She's currently picking up a thread of creative writing and art after a long hiatus due to over-responsibility to everyday life. She lives in Montpelier, Vermont.

TWO POEMS

Jack Foley

MASK

the river is wearing a mask
the trees are wearing masks
the grass has a special separate mask
for each blade
the birds are wearing masks
(look at the cedar waxwings)
houses are wearing masks
there are masks on all the sidewalks
the traffic lights are masked
there are masks on the statues in the cathedral
and on those in the museum
there is a mask over my heart
when I tell you I love you
(but you recognize me)
the streets are wearing masks
(you can hardly make out Brookdale)
all the animals are wearing masks
(look at the bears)
the fish too are masked
as they make their way in the deep

which is also masked
the lone ranger has put a mask on his mask
tonto has been checked for Covid-19
women are wearing masks
their skirts are wearing masks
I see masks on the knees that show
beneath their skirts
I see masks on the snow
covered hills
masks are wearing masks
masquerades are wearing masks
mascara is wearing a mask
mask the knife initially refused
wishing not be regarded as a
common thief
but has finally relented and worn one
and I, as I sit on the rubble of history,
a lone ant on an anthill,
have placed a mask on my book,
on my pen,
on my keyboard
on my computer screen
a mask on my fingers
a mask on my tongue
a mask on my eyes
a mask on my breath
a mask on whatever I have of life

THE BONES OF HISTORY

You try to keep it together
but it gets old and
falls apart.

What was once
in some kind of order
becomes chaos.
You turn your eye away.
Is this what it means
to age?
The world itself
and your country
with a manic, maniac president
at the helm
seems infinitely chaotic
beyond the reach
of even the fiction
of reason.
Was it time
that did this
or constant lack
of attention?
Disease
increases.
Fear
turns to anger
and anger
is everywhere.
These are the bones
of history
not its fruit.
Two thousand years
and we are nowhere.
Full of false creeds
and the disappointment
of friends.

Jack Foley has published 16 books of poetry, 5 books of criticism, a book of stories, and a 1,300-page "chronoencyclopedia," *Visions & Affiliations: California Poetry 1940–2005.* He became well known through his multi-voiced performances with his late wife, Adelle, also a poet. He currently performs with his new life partner, Sangye Land. He has presented poetry on radio station KPFA since 1988 and has received two Lifetime Achievement Awards. A new book of Foley's poetry, *When Sleep Comes: Shillelagh Songs,* has just appeared; and Dana Gioia and Peter Whitfield have edited *Jack Foley's Unmanageable Masterpiece*—a book about Foley's book *Visions & Affiliations.*

COVIDA—MY NEW COMPANION

A Disease of Ruthless Truth

Philippa Rees

I felt her presence the moment she crossed the threshold. I would not claim she "breezed" in, but her penetration came with a cold wind of dread, dread not of illness—nothing in me expected to be one of the chosen—but an unnameable dread that suddenly life as I had known it was to end. It was certain, not apocalyptic.

I should set the chosen victim in context before I introduce you to this ruthless calculating doyenne with her watch chain and gaunt resolve, a Mrs. Danvers mark ten. I was paddling slowly toward old age with some of the irritating symptoms, to which I gave no attention. I still had things to accomplish, a memoir to finish, other works to polish, and the days were filled with purpose and routines. Purpose had driven my puritanical life, to contribute something of small significance. I had long been indifferent to my appearance, or clothes, and I wanted little. I hardly saw anyone. A reason to keep writing was all there was, and it was enough for some to say, "You don't seem anything like eighty." I was nowhere near eighty, then. Three months ago, that "then."

Like any professional invader, Covida cleared her workspace, which was my mind, exterminating any resistance. She knew exactly what was required. I would submit, no nonsense, and since this would be a rehearsal for death I would lie down and sleep while she went about eliminating the value of anything I had achieved, chopping down and uprooting before the pyre of correction consumed it all; the garden of my life lived. All illusions were swept away by her broom of unvarnished truth.

I slept uninterrupted for eight days and eight nights, only broken by a glass held to my lips every four hours, but the inner journey I took was her prelude for the other still to come.

First the landscape went pewter and metallically grey, and the maw of a funnel sucked me slowly and inexorably toward it, until I fell, like Alice into a wonderland of bleak revelations. Grey flattened replicas of Covids floated past, like blood platelets or planarias with their characteristic spikes, as though suspended in a viscous medium, not threatening because being omnipotent they had no need for menace. They were masters in the medium of my blood and brain, and they were a tribe that had total possession, make no mistake.

Then, one at a time, I floated down past recent friends, and each was wrapped in a colored film of slight color, blue or green or grey. I saw that film as my projected imprisonment of those friends by my hopes and expectations of them. Those friends, wrapped like mummies, had never been fully seen because I had projected upon them roles that answered to me. My longing for a reader had failed to differentiate between someone who admired my writing—in sich—from *what* I was writing, which she couldn't believe in, not really. Since the substance of what I was writing was my memories reconstructed with all their innocence, not believing them was not believing in my world or my integrity. So my friendship built over years lay shattered. My hope had blinded me and imprisoned her. So it was with each of them. Another, much younger, was wrapped in my confidence that she had never seen me other than as a contemporary, but Covida ripped off that mask and showed her as kind but never carelessly equal. I wanted her youth and I had expropriated her kindness. I will miss them but one cannot unsee what one has seen.

Covida is a ruthless excavator of truth, the truth about oneself.

After the pewter funnel of recent life, I landed in a black landscape in which the setting sun was a thin sliver of light on the horizon. It had the atmosphere of a Caspar David Friedrich painting, bleak but inevitable. That light was the remnant of my future life, if I was to live. I took a vow, then and there, that if I survived I would not return to the unthinking, semi-conscious existence I had been living. Nor reclothe myself in self-importance, although now the air blows cold about me. How will I spend my days?

I have not yet found another life to live. Perhaps when Covida gives her consent to let me walk more than three hundred yards without staggering, and remain vertical for a whole day, I will. She is parsimonious with her spoonfuls of stamina. Some mornings I rise with a teaspoonful that will last until noon, other days she is liberal with enough to see me through until tea time, and I have fed the dog before the desperation to lie down.

Being stripped naked of all clothes of self-belief, all the satisfactions from accomplishments (and I had a few), leaves little from which to restructure a new existence. Perhaps a dulling of Covida's influence will tempt me to return to smug satisfaction. I hope I will resist.

I have long had a place I go to in the imagination, a weather-beaten grey wooden shack above a cove, shining like a coin, enfolded by the arms of the earth, and known only to gulls. That is where I hope to find a new life. Needing and wanting nothing.

I do wonder whether my single experience is also to be the collective consequence of Covida's invasion of the planet. Will it strip us collectively naked to repent of our blindness? Will we find its ruthless truth cleansing? I give Covida a female gender since women have a deeper appetite for truth, and are more deeply mired in roles that imprison them and those they serve.

Humanity has received new vision, and been stripped of outworn illusions. We, Covida's elected front runners, may have the wind of that in our nostrils. The haltings of the following tribe are still attempting to reduce the sharp salted new air to the recycled old paradigms—"only a kind of flu," "a variant of SARS"—in the hope of holding onto hope that Man has seen this before, and survived. Survived for another chance at mistaken identity and the death of value and values.

The lens of my encounter with her suggested something utterly unique, and ruthlessly intelligent, something impenetrable beneath the superficial symptoms of her presence. The "bends" in which I lurch are appropriate for the depths from which I have risen. She robbed me of every conviction that I knew myself (and I have spent a lifetime following Socrates in that pursuit). The onion has no limits. Nor does the onion of this blundering humanity concerned with appearances, with acquisition, with color and distinctions, with sex and the liberation from gender, in the absurd belief that the individual is thereby defined.

The marvel of the unique individual remains hidden by the fluttering of banners. The Cause obscures the Universal.

PHILIPPA REES has published two works of poetic narrative. *Involution—An Odyssey Reconciling Science to God,* was the product of her experiences and posits the idea that experiential memory is encoded. The history of science has been through the incremental recovery of memory, the major nodes being the insights of genius. Yet science has relegated inspiration to intellectual understanding and created the gulf between it and the spiritual. The other work, a poetic fictional novella, *A Shadow in Yucatan,* paints a portrait of the optimism of the sixties, and its disappointing dissipation. Other published works have been short stories. She has just completed a memoir outlining the experiences that led to *Involution.* She lives in Somerset, UK.

TODAY IS THE DAY

Emily Shurr

We're in it, folks. We're all the way in it.

This is Revelations, this is the Rapture, this is the New Heaven and the New Earth. Old wheels are broken, new wheels are turning, the wheel-within-the-wheel of old is real. This is the collapse of timelines: Look around you. What was projected to happen in decades is now happening in weeks.

In every psyche across the world, in our governments and institutions, our education system, industries, banking, manufacturing, distribution, our climate, our biology, and especially our culture: All are undergoing rapid transformation on the order of a Z-Axis, a new dimension in history. An entirely new and uncharted impulse is being introduced right now, one that could not be predicted or anticipated, one that only existed in the mind of the "true believer," the mystic, and the tech CEO sitting in the desert taking massive doses of psychedelics.

Now is the time: Our work to re-enchant the world (sing a new song, build a new life together) is urgently, even desperately needed. We must be bold now. Unafraid of emerging into our wholeness, undeterred from sharing our greatest gifts. Our skills, our vision, our insight, our care, our writing, our stories, our love.

This is the Great Shakedown.

For once the scientists and astrologers, the ancients and the futurists agree. This time is truly without precedent: The inflection points of history may have felt this seismic, but never has the scale been so large or the effects so ubiquitous.

The crisis *is* the gift. The pain *is* the opportunity.

Release the ways that keep us stuck, our voices stifled, our spirits cramped and afraid.

Are we victims, permanently withdrawn, subject to greed and control? Or are we flowing forward with inner knowing, creators of sane and loving new models of work and family and community, guided by mutual aid and shared responsibility, determining our own course? We are deciding right now—and we keep on deciding every day.

And! We are not flipping the script, making the old victims into the new oppressors. We are writing a whole new story.

We are praying and writing and teaching and telling and visioning and crafting new worlds into being.

NO ONE CAN DO THIS ALONE. We need each other.

And the good news is—we HAVE each other!

EMILY SHURR works as a coach for neurodiversity, spiritual emergence, and end-of-life counseling. She is a consultant to Fortune 100s, government agencies, and innovative education programs, and an initiated Shakta Tantrick with roots in French Existentialism and Celtic Catholicism. She holds a master's degree in religion (medical ethics) from Yale Divinity School and a B.A. in religious studies from the University of Tennessee.

MOVING FORWARD . . .

How Do We Get Out of This One?

Richard Grossinger

I. ITS HOUR COME ROUND

Now that we are in corona time, there are no rules, deadlines, or endgame. We are playing on the virus' terms while maintaining a panacealike casuistry, hoping that the previous world was a real one and this is a limited interlude. But we have come to an Ides in history, in human life on a planet (Gaia) orbiting a sun-star (Sol). Climate may be the planet's real Ides, but the virus is an envoy. Climate is corona at a planetary scale. Forget sheltering at home. Earth is home. There is no second home.

COVID-19 evinces Earth's biological resilience, not the resilience we prize but one as microbial as our pre-Cambrian biome—a hermetic underbelly to the Anthropocene as current as the Wuhan market and as old as the first cave images. It is like World War II in scope but deeper and without ordnance or battlefield drama. It is like an asteroid hit but of subtle energy rather than fire and dust. As it deletes familiar strata and melts time like a Salvador Dali clock, days take weeks or sometimes years to pass in a bardo state that is neither quite waking nor dream. Each day is totally different; each day, we are different. In another sense, time seems to be running backwards or in simultaneous tracks.

Any song or movie, book or dance from before COVID-19 has changed its energy, picked up sci-fi surrealism and a precognitive tinge.

COVID marks the end of transhumanism. We are *part* of the ecosphere. We can try to flee it on devices, but any real escape requires such a technological leap and shift of belief that our attempts to date have produced only hell realms. The goal of consciousness singularity in software—AI replacing people—is as psychotic and phantasmal as that of colonizing the galaxy.

COVID-19 is Cassandra *and* Paul Revere: "Creatures of water and air! You have another course. And it may not be too late."

COVID marks the end of tribal ideology. By scrambling tribes and ideologies, it tells us to seek common ground because, from its standpoint, we *are* common ground. It also tells us we cannot be ruled by Babel—disinsformation and evangelism—because we then can speak neither to it nor ourselves.

COVID marks the end of American exceptionalism. That goes without saying.

COVID has *everything* to say about nuclear winter without mentioning it at all.

When gods and goddesses speak, as nature or as themselves, we are called to a new dreamtime: the garden and hunt and weir before the lords of hydraulic civilization saw an opening and turned it into Sumer, Egypt, and patriarchy for the next six thousand years. But six millennia, even with accumulated bricks, mortar, and silicon grids, are a sliver of a Holocene kalpa.

An anarchy of freedom is emerging: cooperation across societal barriers, neighborhood solidarity against the state. Hospitals and grocery stores have become hospices, temples, non-cash economies, as people create pods or arks to get themselves out of central control—of food, of energy, of the ownership of labor, of the arbitration of life, death, and the afterlife.

Backlash too: in Hong-Kong, Nigeria, India, Yemen, Khazakhstan, Rio.

The priest has left the altar, and *"the rough beast, its hour come round at last,"* has begun to take a form. It is what we dreaded and what we have been waiting for.

Don't say why did it have to be this, why did we have to be awakened in this way? You know and I know, we wouldn't have listened to anything less. We wouldn't have stopped our markets and bling and *mishigas* without a warning shot that got our attention.

Dead refugee children washing ashore in Greece and Texas didn't do it. Hiroshima didn't do it. The *Interahamwe* and Islamic State and Syrian War didn't do it. The Cuban Crisis and Vietnam and Iraq Wars didn't do it. 9/11 and Al Qaeda didn't do it.

Evolutionary astrologer Laurie Matsue writes, "2020 is like the world is in an ayahuasca ceremony together—and most people have neither prepared for it nor do they even know they're in it and there's no shaman. The shaman is meant to create some containment around the energy of the ceremony, and there's definitely none of that going on."

2. GAME SHOW

No one knows what's really going on. Highly informed dives into COVID-ness yield diametrically opposed reports, explanations, warnings, complaints, shamings, and prescriptions. Some people question its very existence or at least the risk of deadly harm to themselves; they don't know anyone who has gotten sick. It's a parallel reality from which they are magically or socioeconomically exempted, until suddenly they can't breathe, and others around them are sick.

The virus has been muddled by conflicting information, contradictory theories and assumptions, and clashes of political, meta-political, and social attitudes, motives, and agendas. There is no *truth-du-jour,* let alone a clear long-term picture. Narratives of denial spawn under propaganda-driven governances and hierarchies of newspeak as well as the designed counterproductivity of the system (hospitals, medical manufacturers, insurance pyramids, pharmaceutical companies, supply chains, banks, federal reserves).

For Donald Trump the world is sourced in a game show and his own ratings—there is no competing value. The buck never stops; there are just more contestants and hoopla. In a landscape of make-believe, interchangeable realities, where pleasure has been reduced to either malignant narcissism or a victory over someone else, the kill rate of COVID-19 is, at worst, collateral damage. As Joseph Stalin is said to have said: "A single death is a tragedy; a million deaths is a statistic."

"Trumpism" is an invulnerable prosperity cult and Republican ghost dance. The coronavirus "cannot" exist (or be a real threat), thus it *does not* exist as such or is not dangerous. An inflated flu, a rogue statistic, a manipulated "plandemic" infects people under aliases. Morbidity and death become fake news, political sublimations.

The neologism "plandemic" (false pandemic) is adopted by polar factions—on one side, Second Amendment irregulars, QAnon devotees, Proud Boys, and biblical fundamentalists; on the other, anarchists, Pharma foes, energy healers, and Antifa. They are not only polar to each other but internally *bi*polar, inflating and deflating their own credos in manic-depressive bursts that mimic arcs of loyalty. The Right scapegoats the Deep State, a globalist conspiracy, and George Soros; the Left blames transnational corporations, Nazi science, and Bill Gates.

The Right embraces mob neo-paganism, the Second Coming, and the next Aryan demagogue.

The Left is "woke" with ideological scientism, faux compassion, and moral self-righteousness, which feels a whole lot like morality.

The claim that Government infectious-disease czar Anthony Fauci created COVID-19 in a Chinese lab is a "plandemic" of both the Right and the Left—the Left for anti-corporate reasons, the Right for anti-Fauci reasons.

Microbiological, epidemiological, and demographic mysteries have been conflated with proselytizing obfuscations and mal- and meta-information such that their threads are now inextricably entangled. In the absence of a "people's" science, there is no baseline or veridicality.

The discrepancy between places that *should* be overrun with COVID-19 and those that actually are—as well as between those exposed and those who get sick or horrifically sick or become asymptomatically infected (or even what asymptomatic infection or contagion mean)—leaves plausible deniability for just about any position while posing unsolved riddles of a "novel coronavirus."

Sweden's rejection of sheltering in place has been, at once, a singular success of herd immunity and a disaster of runaway contagion. Opposite interpretations of the same script perform on the same stage in the same theater.

Prior exposure to other coronaviruses is thought to have enhanced some people's immunity to COVID-19. Conversely, prior exposure has led to a cytokine storm and collapse of the immune system, perhaps the case with patients who start to recover from COVID and suddenly end up on ventilators—likewise with those exposed to cyclical but less serious flus before the 1918 Spanish variant; they fared worse for the same reason. Legitimate, though discredited, scientific studies now indicate that standard flu vaccines make recipients *more* susceptible to coronaviruses and with more deadly outcomes.

The dilemma goes beyond COVID's back loop of belief systems, safety parameters, and lifestyles or its uncertainty states of particle output, aerosol half-life, and RNA content. We are metaphysically trapped, between climate change and capital growth, vaccines and immune responses, materiality of UFOs and inhabitability of Mars. Markets are up, but money buys less, so they keep printing it. Eventually it will turn into something else, or something else will become money.

As deadly, invasive, and insidiously self-camouflaging as the coronavirus is, it has become a cover story for other long-incubating crises and miasms of our civilization.

Nipah, a paramyxovirus, has a 40–75 percent human kill rate based on the worst outcomes of 250 employees infected in 1999 on a large pig farm at the edge of a rainforest in Malaysia. The captive pigs feasted on rotting date-palm fruits and mangos covered with bat saliva, so the virus got assistance in double-jumping species, foregoing a few centuries of intermediate incubation. Aside from a hundred or so unfortunate workers, the civilized world dodged a bullet, one of *known* curbed outbreaks since the late nineties (MERS, SARS, ebola, and avian and swine flus included).

3. ALL OTHER WARS

COVID struck at the weakest seams holding society's myths and legends *as if* together. The scales are not just out of balance; they are no longer scales.

When monetization of value replaces freedom, spiritual freedom, and meaningfulness, the West has fallen under a Soviet-style lockdown far more deadly and devious than a military dictatorship or a coronavirus. There is no need for armies; the people have enslaved themselves, including with their own Second-Amendment-guaranteed assault rifles. The prison is the mind; its bars include the notion that fun is quantifiable and that restoring the flow of goods means restoring happiness and normality.

"I can't breathe!" had the force of overlapping pandemics. The irony bore a brutally un-ironic message. Whether the smothering agent was external, casually cruel, and racist or internal, parasitic, and impersonal, victims were being choked to death.

Eventually melting glaciers will drown the continents. Before that, toxins from the continents will choke coral reefs and sea life. *Nothing* will be able to breathe. The great forests, the lungs of the Earth, are being attacked as well.

Freedom of movement, personal safety, economic well-being, careers, physical intimacy, longstanding hopes and plans, the amelioration of suffering and grief are drowned in not just social distancing and fear of the virus but division and isolation: hyperconsumerism breeding hyperindividualism.

Spaciousness and freedom of speech are stifled by self-righteous indignation, authoritarian reductionism, and language police. Holistic doctor Sarah Kent writes, "The COVID response makes us all vectors of infection, potential poisoners of the masses just by breathing, let alone by disseminating our seditious views on life, the universe, and everything. How have we all been dehumanized to the point of being lethal vectors in each others' universes?"

In New York, St. Paul, Los Angeles, Philadelphia, Oakland, and elsewhere, protests against police brutality and institutionalized racism escalated beyond liberal fallbacks of social justice and reparation—to looting the malls of the empire with their Atlantean-like crypts. New York's Fifth Avenue and Beverly Hills' Rodeo Drive were smashed open, picked clean. Mobs chanting "Eat the Rich!" and "Hit a Mothafucka!" also burned down Oglala and Ojibwa museums and youth centers in Minneapolis and St. Paul. The fire knew no philosophy at Alexandria; it did not read Parmenides or Plato, only the elemental structure of worlds that were, worlds that were to come.

The revolution against property, civil order, and the imagination has been camouflaged by a Trumpian republic of wealth, pomp, and power. Under that mirage, home invasion will be as fashionable in Los Angeles and Houston as in Baghdad or Tegucigalpa.

The deeper impact of COVID-19 is the vulnerability of our brief Holocene symposium of democracy and art. Seattle's Capitol Hill Autonomous Zone was not Woodstock—love, peace, and cosmos. CHAZ was a Burning Man free-crime zone, a statehood away (Texas? California? New Mexico?) from fentanyl and methamphetamine trade routes—as if the stupid wall will keep out what it is inside.

Opportunism reigns, armed robberies in downtown San Francisco and New York's Upper East Side. Those same mobs—Right or Left hardly matters—will sack Trump Tower, Mar-a-Lago, Wal-Mart, and Microsoft *before* the flood. Libya is not as far from Miami as it is from Alpha Centauri.

Yesterday it was the Islamic State destroying idols, churches, mosques, and neighborhoods of Mosul and Aleppo, the remnants of Zoroastrian/Sufi civilization. Tomorrow it will be the French

Revolution and Red Guards in Boston and Baton Rouge. COVID-19 could be the last bell before open sea.

Between Bob Dylan's 1962 "A Hard Rain's a-Gonna Fall" and David Bowie's 1972 "Cygnet Committee" (*And I want to believe / In the madness that calls 'Now'*) there was still world enough and time.

4. VAMPIRES

COVID-19 has changed in four months from a respiratory condition and mock flu to a blood malignancy, a far scarier proposition given the thoughtforms and dark goddess behind bat-vampire transmutation. The undead are sucking not just iron-binding essence but vital force out of those closest to them, and their incubi are barely .1 micron long. They are no longer bats, but they come from bats. Clusters fall ill in waves, deteriorate with astonishing swiftness, drag themselves to hospitals from different sites in unison, looking like the victims of voodoo, their hair standing up, dazed expressions on their faces. The disease is accompanied by lucid dreams, guided trances, out-of-body travel, precognition, ancestral visitation, time-space distortions, hypnagogia.

A thirty-year-old Swedish martial artist in good health, after contracting the virus reported a feeling like being waterboarded, buried alive and revived, again and again. Every organ hurt. In warning others not to take COVID lightly, he messaged, "It's as if there is something intelligent inside me that's trying to kill me. An evil entity, a poison, something conscious that's torturing me from within."

It's a monstropedia of orcs, werewolves, and corpses in Black Death piles and refrigeration trucks.

The virus is the unseen real, masquerading as symptoms and sentences, choosing its victims with precise yet arbitrary criteria; it is at once as horrifically thorough, metastasizing, and fatal as AIDS or cancer and as glancing as a cold and headache. How do the Three Fates cut their thread so unevenly?

When the commodity of the health system fails, the nature of death changes. When the nature of death changes, the nature of life changes. A life that is no longer insurable against death or poverty (or discard) devolves to Medieval-like expendability—and witchcraft. Meanwhile, death is left to speak for itself, to the dead.

The medical system has no pills or potions, no silver bullet or golden stake.

Hematologically, COVID pathology introduces a platelet-clotting factor relative to age, sex, race, ethnicity, and blood type—in a range of studies, those with A antigens are apparently more susceptible, those without (O positive or negative) thirty-five to fifty percent less. (In other studies, blood types B and AB are more susceptible, while A is neutral.)

Apparently, COVID-19 spikes bind angiotensin-converting enzyme (ACE2) receptors of endothelial cells, leading to local inflammation of the walls of blood vessels and capillaries, raising blood pressure and causing clotting and organ failure. The symptoms looked respiratory at first because of not only precursor flu-like templates but entrance through the nose, mouth, eyes, and throat, binding alveolocytes lining the lungs, leading to an auto-immune coagulation and a change of lipid metabolism. Increased fatty-acid accumulation meant difficulty breathing. From there, it spread to other organs.

Ventilators were an understandably mistaken intervention.

5. A STATISTIC FOR EVERY BELIEF SYSTEM

How does one explain seemingly healthy young people who undergo multiple organ failure, while others, including statistically more vulnerable folks, remain asymptomatic after exposure? Or how did a healthy thirty-year-old who practiced social distancing and didn't know how he got exposed contract such a severe form of COVID-19 that he suffered heart and lung failure, mini-strokes, and the prospect of amputation before succumbing, while a sixty-year-old showed no ill effects despite multiple exposures at indoor gatherings? Why does the virus explode in some places, stay confined in others, and cross only some geographies?

Even those who are asymptomatic, apparently the majority, carry a stowaway in their organisms, and there is no telling what shingles-like expression waits down-century. . . .

Who gets sick, how sick, and for how long, and who tests positive, are a consequence of multiple co-factors, including intensity and virulence of exposure, natural immunity, inherited enzymatic combinations, diet, body weight, underlying morbidity, adherence to social distancing and face-masking, and countless hidden variables, some of them at a cell and subcell level, others psychic, quantum, cultural, symbolic, psychosomatic, and paraphysical. Some strains are apparently more contagious than others, leading to super-spreader events from asymptomatic carriers. Despite a steady stream of out-of-state summer visitors to Maine, the state's viral load remained low until a single wedding at an inn in Millinocket led to twenty-two new primary cases, fourteen secondary hosts, and twenty-four tertiary hosts carrying the disease quickly more than a hundred miles, including to a prison and nursing home. Contact tracing shows a geography as Newtonian as the path of a hurricane.

Mask-wearing, social distancing, and tracking of those who test positive are a *sine qua non* to slow the spread of COVID-19, for years if necessary. There is no other exit strategy.

At the same time, the virus is a cover for surveillance, totalitarian technocracy, and centralized power. From tracking by cell signal, 'bot implant, or facial recognition will come denial of entry to stores and homes without a Pharma chip or certificate of RNA mod. We end up in both *1984* and *Brave New World,* locked down and sedated. If you want to control the masses, what better way than to require they be inoculated and medicated—diagnosed, pathologized, and rendered correctable by a providential bounty of transhumanist science. Orwellian vaccines that keep people from benign ones make a rote rejection of the anti-vax position *even more* anti-vax.

Forget paranoid anti-government myths about masks and vaccines as a first stage of corporate control. That's street kitsch. There are three wars going on with overlapping battlefields. The first is the most visible one, where I cast a daily vote. It is the hospital workers, physicians, nurses, grocery-store workers, bus drivers, teachers, and the vulnerable, poor, and innocent against Second Amendment bullies, White supremacists, climate-change and virus deniers, tithing abundance cults masquerading as churches, survivalist militias, and fascist exceptionalists.

I also cast my daily vote with the second: healers, herbalists, shamans, and a few old-fashioned pragmatic family doctors against the medical industrial complex with its shareholders, lobbyists, agitprop, and bought politicians.

When competing realities are valid in different ways, we need rational, trustworthy leaders to cut the Gordian knot. Instead, we have hooligans exploiting cognitive dissonance.

These battlefields disguise a third and most dangerous war. It is all of humanity, including most of the oligarchs (the Trump family too), remaining Indigenous tribes and elders, scientists, the rich, the poor, and the homeless against a scourge and deep state so extra-judicial and unassailable—such a master of dissensions and disguises—that even COVID-19 palls before it. The crisis is, we don't know and are not being allowed to find out; instead, we turn against one another while the real oligarchs build climate shelters and biospheres thousands of feet below the topsoil.

As Diane di Prima wrote centuries ago, "The war that matters is the war against the imagination—all other wars are subsumed in it."

6. THE END OF THE PLAGUE

COVID-19 will end only with a vaccine (as polio did), a treatment for those inflicted (like HIV), or herd immunity.

Or, COVID-19 will simply dissipate.

Let's distinguish Donald Trump's disingenuous or delusional

agitprop from rosier assessments of the coronavirus' possible futures. The notion that it will just go away is based on a number of different belief systems, not all of them secular. The scientific prognoses invoke COVID's natural, non-correcting RNA mutations.

But many scientists believe that the virus may self-select for *greater* contagion and virulence under the same Darwinian parameters. Others say that no natural pathogenic virus becomes more virulent.

Either way, COVID is a serial shape-shifter.

Since the virus camouflages itself and tricks cells into believing its RNA is theirs, delaying an immune response while it replicates, T-cell (white blood cell) backup is critical in the context of vaccine-triggered immune response. Herd immunity, itself a widely misunderstood and misapplied concept, relies on sustained antibody immunity and a vaccine, neither of which is guaranteed. In fact, numerous cases of apparent re-infection suggest that antibody protection wanes, if it develops at all, after a month or two with a cardiovascular coronavirus. There are no antibody-based "immunity passports," meaning no guaranteed exit strategy.

The ideal vaccine, its development accelerated by unprecedented international cooperation, electron microscopes, nanotechnology, polymer enhancement, and computer modeling, also overlooks that scientists do not understand the virus' mechanism, how it makes itself a mockingbird in cells and differentially affects tissues, or the depth of its own capacity to learn and change.

Molecular biologists do not know what will decoy COVID-19 across its spectrum—lungs, heart, kidneys, neurons, toes—nor how to sustain such an effect without continual revaccination. The out-of-nowhere Russian vaccine (August 2020), rogue in terms of WHO protocols yet endorsed by Vladimir Putin to the extent that his daughter was inoculated, is either a mirage and a fraud or a low-risk socialist medicine, offered to the world for free, to combat the RNA-infiltrating serums being developed by capitalist labs and governments.

The most promising isopaths, made from other hominid coronaviruses, steal instructions for COVID-19's Trojan-horse spike and disguising enzyme and induce antibody and T-cell responses. Two unusual llama antibody fragments (nanobodies) also block COVID's spike glycoproteins from binding to the ACE2 receptors.

But there is always the possibility of *introducing* even deadlier agents, a gambit we seem willing to turn over, with no liability, to the polities that brought us Vioxx and opioids. There is a reason that it takes fifty years to develop a benign vaccine.

Maybe this time will be different, with the whole world watching the corner-cutting and risk assessments. Maybe this time will be different with the best and brightest of a rainbow planet watching not only corporate thugs and professional liars but one another. Maybe this time we will get a vaccine at the depth and wisdom of our lineage—a Bach and da Vinci, a Coltrane and Baryshnikov of vaccines—and no one will get autism or chronic fatigue or mercury poisoning or COVID-19. We will get a vaccine of compassion rather than profit, of communion rather than exile, of love. Maybe. Because when the asteroid comes or another three degrees Fahrenheit heat the pot, it's going to raze everything, wipe the slate clean, of dinosaurs too.

The real gold standard of a treatment's effectiveness is prevention or cure under game conditions—unexplainable intercessions allowed— not performance against a placebo in a static simulation in which factors of transference, projection, and empathic participation, let alone dynamic molecular quantifications and other quanta, have been ignored or inadvertently canceled or purged. Living systems are superpositional, transmutational, shamanic, homeopathic, and paraphysically entangled. That can't always be replicated artificially in a trial.

The trouble is, biochemists still don't understand the vital force, the memory of water, telekinesis, potentization, synchronicity, vibration, prayer, placebo, thoughtforms, holism, the power of similars and sigils, the difference between healing and hexing, nonlinear effects, and the nano underground—or even why an allopathic isopath developed by AstraZeneca or Moderna should be better protection than a COVID-19 nosode potentized homeopathically from a microdose of viral sputum.

A vaccine has to whack every mole and cover every gap and spike like Aesop's wind trying to blow a man's coat off. A nosode only has to be like the sun and smile; its radiance goes everywhere.

No treatment, vaccine, or intervention, however, will restore the old order or its economy or society. We have made entry into the next world age, Aquarian in an intrinsic sense, and we will arrive there only because we have no way back.

In her 2006 book *End of Days,* psychic Sylvia Browne predicted that "a severe pneumonia-like illness" would appear suddenly around the year 2020. It would sweep the globe before disappearing mysteriously, reappearing ten years later before vanishing for good.

Despite critiques of this particular precognition and psychic formulation in general, and minor inaccuracies of prognostication, Browne's omen is still in play—clairvoyant basics.

7. TREATMENTS

It is possible that COVID-19 is containable before it gets into the bloodstream and wreaks havoc with cells and organs. If so, ninety-nine percent of the people infected could stop it at the level of a flu. Alternative prevention methods and cures range from the COVID-19 nosode to various herbs, mushrooms, cultured vegetables, kimchi, vitamins, red algae, minerals (colloidal silver, zinc, magnesium), hyperbaric oxygen, etc. The seaweed extract RPI-27 (named after Rensselaer Polytechnic Institute) attached to the COVID-19 spike and outperformed remdesivir (which is more a last-ditch palliative than a medicine with its own Hippocratic wisdom).

In many cases, the positive effect is too complex and multivariate to pin down.

It is worth querying the most controversial pharmaceutical. Despite Donald Trump and Jair Bolsonaro's bent for subversive make-believe, many reputable doctors claim to be using hydroxychloroquine (or chloroquine) with total to partial success for both prevention and treatment of COVID-19. One interpretation is that its lysosome-penetrating activity slows antigen production and enhances autophagy—cellular cleansing of its own cytoplasm.

Other herbalists and doctors, plus most physicians, say that hydroxychloroquine is useless or worse. I will make the counter case not necessarily to persuade you (or even me) but as a thought experiment:

Hydroxychloroquine's clinical-trial "failures" include excessive doses (2.4 g in the first 24 hours, 800 mg/day after!), tests on hospitalized patients too sick to benefit, failure to use any of the medical combinations known to activate or catalyze hydroxychloroquine (zinc is a molecular complement to most cell-vector reactions)—then international pressure on physicians to stop prescribing, aggressive cutting off of supplies, the touting of advances on the savior vaccine and expensive non-generic drugs like remdesivir, inflating its more meager benefits; then media hysteria, censorship, ridicule, and gaslighting every time hydroxychloroquine is positively advanced by Donald Trump or one of his lackeys, *as if biochemical properties of the drug itself had become synonymous with Trump's ignorance, pandering, and magical thinking.* (M.D. Meryl Nass says, "In the U.S., 'Never Trump' morphed into 'Never Hydroxychloroquine," and the result for the pandemic is 'Never Over.'")

A generic, inexpensive drug, prescribed safely for sixty-five years to millions of patients, has been declared dangerous for COVID-19 alone. Yet once double-blind, double-bind protocols are removed, people are apparently cured by hydroxychloroquine. NYU and Henry Ford hospitals (New York City and Detroit) report fifty percent reduction in deaths. Similarly without clinical explanation, homeopathic hospitals during the Spanish flu saw even greater reduction in death rates. Remote reviewing, telepathy, and telekinesis also don't deliver under test conditions.

Hydroxychloroquine raises multiple issue of ethics, conspiracy, and false flag so complicated that it is impossible to tell who the real-stakes players are among medical institutions, pharmaceutical conglomerates, billionaires, and oligarchs. It's even hard to know if *they can tell* because the ones pulling the strings are not the ones driving the authorized pandemic response: those beneficiaries of emergency government programs, banks repossessing real estate, executives and shareholders of pharmaceutical companies, all participating in windfalls without driving them, sometimes while even opposing it. Ninety percent of humanity is caught in this web.

In any case, presidents Trump and Bolsonaro have no trouble obtaining hydroxychloroquine for themselves while promoting it in the context of such delusional and jingoist conceits that they tacitly caricature it. Thrown in with killing the virus by drinking bleach, hydroxychloroquine became one more Trumpian trope rather than a real medicine.

Hydroxychloroquine's supporters also include loonies, occult fabulists, Fox News shills, Trump family sycophants, and other people of the lie. Once the drug got cited as a COVID cure by Houston M.D. Stella Immanuel, an exemplar of magic-think, pop demonology, and cosmic conspiracies, the drug became its own punchline. Her dumbed-down mashups not only led to people conflating the virus with astral sex with demons and witches and alien DNA but also doused serious consideration of the paranormal, the astral realm, spirit energy, or the extraterrestrial origin of DNA. Instead, hydroxychloroquine became a mock cure for sexual witchcraft and alien biotech. Of course, the performance of the medicine and doctoring of this woman have nothing to do with her private cosmology.

The situation shows how powerful and consolidated a hypothetical conspiracy might be, enlisting allies from both sides. Trump has become irrelevant or serves an auxiliary strategy of extending the pandemic and consolidating oligarchic power at a level above his own meager empire—again, not tweeted "population control" memes but a technocratically driven agenda at a *Star Wars* scale, an unknown control and power so hegemonous and Sauron-like that it pulls the strings of the CDC, WHO, Amazon.com, Google, Microsoft, Facebook, Twitter, Instagram, the Saudis and Chinese, Republicans and Democrats alike. Whether it is of common Earth or not, it has left a material presence. We are all at risk.

But is this kabuki dance even happening, or is it another psychotic fantasy of a world on the brink? (Meryl Nass's anthraxvaccine blogspot is a fair starting point.)

8. THE ORIGIN AND DESTINY OF COVID-19

Mainstream microbiologists and virologists have "proven" both that COVID-19 *had to have been* bioengineered (chimerical spikes and Fibonacci sequences) and that it *could not have been* bioengineered (96.2 percent similarity to a SARS-like virus in bat feces from Yunnan's Shitou Cave and no known close-to-near lab correlates). Those who believe that it was bioengineered shear between deep cynics who argue that it was released as a bioweapon and mere paranoids who favor accident.

The original bat RNA has added sequences seemingly from HIV that could indicate intentional weaponization or search for an AIDS vaccine gone wrong. In any case, it is weaponized now.

It's not overly "conspiracy theorist" to think that the source lies somewhere in a complicated nexus of events and motives: one researcher brings back the COVID mother and another leaves the lab with her children unknowingly hitching under his fingernails or clinging to a crease in his pants. The pandemic may be an inevitable consequence of Murphy's and Darwin's laws meeting under technocratic hubris—a most unwelcome collaboration.

The issue is not even whether this one came out of the Wuhan lab; it is that, with such labs in existence and multiplying (as they justify their existences by one another), the next one, or the one after it, will.

To even worry about whether COVID-19 escaped (or was set loose) from the Wuhan coronavirus lab, as opposed to arising naturally, is to assume that a verdict of origin means anything more than one raindrop this way or that. It's a jungle regardless, whether it's a rainforest, ocean, single strand of algae or seaweed, water droplet full of rotifers, or a cell. Once nature and culture are entangled, it's all nature (atomic algorithm) or all culture (symbol, sign, contamination). The rusting machine (or cyber-hardware) in the garden is the dandelion or virus growing out of terra-formed trash. The lab is a hominid-infested cave with sophisticated hand-axes and cleavers.

The "bioweapon" cadre differs on whether COVID has been as deadly as planned or a disappointment—that verdict depends on how many and which people (or populations) were supposed to die, and it intersects the hydroxychloroquine controversy on the matter of whom the drug was *supposed* to protect and whether it has been more or less effective than intended.

Then, among those who believe that COVID-19 crossed naturally from bats and pangolins or by another zoonotic route, there are similar disagreements about whether the virus is now strengthening by natural selection or weakening through routine copying errors and gene drift.

Recent analyses of sewage from Europe and South America dating well before COVID-19 showed up in Wuhan indicate that its agents may have been present throughout the biosphere before being ignited by some environmental factor or population tipping point and/or a heedlessly heightened electromagnetic field (Wuhan's 5G is usually implicated). Once again, natural immunity, habitation clusters, and the bioelectric body play unknown roles in homeostasis, until they don't. Then a case becomes a pandemic.

In a metaphysical context, pathology goes from a warp in the Astral to blocked flow in the Etheric to the body. A Lemurian age replaces modernity.

Yet South Korean and Chinese companies are already well on their way to 6G. Zoom meetings will be fully three-dimensional—holographic. You can examine widgets and walk through each other in virtual rooms like ghosts. The magnified virus, its purple and pink spiked cartoon spheres floating among us like giant balloons, can be examined by scientists in multiple labs at the scale of a liver or, for that matter, an automobile or a star. Tardigrades will collide with bears.

While we create virtual reality, we obliterate vital streams that have methodically, over billions of years, seined a path for our souls to *embody*.

Physician Zach Bush has derived a complex counter-narrative around the virus, concluding with the most optimistically liberating diagnosis. I can't do justice to his system here, nor can I square it with other corona information and lore. Like many things about this pandemic, it floats somewhere among new science, viral meta-linguistics, environmental tipping points, and mythology in the sense that our myths are ahead of our facts (they have more paradox-capable gigabytes). In my super-condensation of Bush's scenario, viruses and retroviruses, from the beginning of life on Earth, transport RNA within microbiomes. They are natural genetic updating machines. Without ancient viruses, our cells could not have developed stem pluripotency nor would mammals and primates have evolved. Alleles jumping species and phyla is what led to the differentiation of the original blastula. RNA from insects, spiders, algae, club mosses, and octopi has infiltrated our lineage—we are viral and pandemic in our database.

The modern world has triggered a radical transformation of our microbiome. COVID-19's new RNA spike is a commensurate reading of pesticides in the agricultural industry (notably Monsanto's Roundup with glyphosate, which literally kills the soil), antibiotics pumped into the sad captives of factory farms (particularly pigs as they exude lake-size cesspools), air pollution (disgorges of methane, carbon dioxide, and particulate matter), and a pharmaceuticalized world.

Clumping with these various toxins, COVID-19 runs far too much information through our microbiome. This overload, not the virus, is what is making people sick and killing them. The hypoxia of COVID is not a classic respiratory symptom but cyanide poisoning in keeping with the climate crisis, air and soil pollution, and reduction of planetary oxygen. It is a hyperinflammatory immune response or cytokine storm from increased neurotransmission between cells.

Yet, according to Bush, most of those infected have their RNA updated without serious harm. From his outlier view, our species is responding to its altered planet by changing its microbiome, so the pandemic is a biological awakening, species metamorphosis, and healing crisis. It will result in a new species, in a physical or a subtle body.

A vaccine will likely not alleviate the pandemic or restore the old order, it will only add to toxic informational overload. Again, one dude's revelation.

The thing about myths is that they can be true in the deepest sense but take hundreds, thousands, or tens of thousands of years to manifest. Bush's COVID loses scale and verisimilitude in a crowded hospital of the dying in Houston or Miami.

Some psychics believe that there is more than one virus or something else is also making people sick. The balance of the atmosphere, its vibration, has been thrown off by chemtrails, HAARP (high-frequency active auroral research program interference), or Elon Musk's Falcon 9 rocket punching a 560-mile-hole in the ionosphere. Yeah, it healed. Gigantic Jupiter (1,321.3 times the volume of Earth) healed the black nuclear cloud from NASA detonating the *Galileo* spacecraft in its atmosphere, but the explosion changed Jovian astrology *forever.*

Victims of COVID-19 have the bends as if they are coming up from the Pacific Ocean floor or climbing Mount Everest because the distortion in the air has gotten into their cells—their pressure chambers responding to the pressure chamber of the planet itself.

My sense is that COVID cast a shadow before it arrived, a deepening hollow that formed roughly between the election of Donald Trump and the fires of Australia—a boom economy that felt like anything but. Astrologers kept saying that they could feel something else there but they didn't know what it was, though it kept getting vaster and emptier, camouflaged by a dazzle and glut of platforms. Pastoral and romantic texture were being drained from the world and replaced by an artificially sweetened, deficit-generated substitute.

Six friends of mine, separated by age, geography, belief system, and how I know them, died prematurely or mysteriously in the last two years, as if they were getting out before the trouble. No one here sees the big picture. I certainly don't.

The real battle, the big one, beyond even COVID, beyond race and gender, is for our souls, our hearts, the natural world, and the bardos of life and death.

The chaos magicians didn't win World War II—we came together once, even the ostensibly vanquished, to promote progressive democracy and freedom. They have returned with a more effective game plan. Getting out of this trap will require our best shamans and witches as well as true scientists and honest governments.

COVID-19 is a magician (Tarot Trump One) who hasn't begun to reveal her slips and sleights, but future worlds depend on learning her magic and making her our ally among the other microbes and spirit guides in our biome. As at 9/11 we have also drawn Trump Sixteeen: a Tower struck by lightning, falling figures of a suddenly obsolete reality. Trump Seventeen is The Star, an androgyne dipping in the waters of unknown worlds and suns.

AUGUST 2020

RICHARD GROSSINGER is the curator of Sacred Planet Books for Inner Traditions. He is the cofounder and former publisher of North Atlantic Books. With a Ph.D. in ecological anthropology from the University of Michigan, Grossinger has written widely acclaimed books on alternative medicine, cosmology, embryology, and consciousness, including *Bottoming Out the Universe: Why There Is Something Rather Than Nothing* (Inner Traditions, 2020). His main psychospiritual practices have been dreams and symbols, *t'ai chi ch'uan*, craniosacral therapy, and the Sethian system of psychic energy taught by John Friedlander and Gloria Hemsher.

INDEX